AF843844

ENDOCRINOLOGY RESEARCH AND CLINICAL DEVELOPMENTS

BIOMEDICAL OSTEOPOROSIS TREATMENT

ENDOCRINOLOGY RESEARCH AND CLINICAL DEVELOPMENTS

Additional books in this series can be found on Nova's website under the Series tab.

Additional e-books in this series can be found on Nova's website under the e-book tab.

ENDOCRINOLOGY RESEARCH AND CLINICAL DEVELOPMENTS

BIOMEDICAL OSTEOPOROSIS TREATMENT

MASAYOSHI YAMAGUCHI

NOVA BIOMEDICAL

New York

Copyright © 2013 by Nova Science Publishers, Inc.

All rights reserved. No part of this book may be reproduced, stored in a retrieval system or transmitted in any form or by any means: electronic, electrostatic, magnetic, tape, mechanical photocopying, recording or otherwise without the written permission of the Publisher.

For permission to use material from this book please contact us:
Telephone 631-231-7269; Fax 631-231-8175
Web Site: http://www.novapublishers.com

NOTICE TO THE READER

The Publisher has taken reasonable care in the preparation of this book, but makes no expressed or implied warranty of any kind and assumes no responsibility for any errors or omissions. No liability is assumed for incidental or consequential damages in connection with or arising out of information contained in this book. The Publisher shall not be liable for any special, consequential, or exemplary damages resulting, in whole or in part, from the readers' use of, or reliance upon, this material. Any parts of this book based on government reports are so indicated and copyright is claimed for those parts to the extent applicable to compilations of such works.

Independent verification should be sought for any data, advice or recommendations contained in this book. In addition, no responsibility is assumed by the publisher for any injury and/or damage to persons or property arising from any methods, products, instructions, ideas or otherwise contained in this publication.

This publication is designed to provide accurate and authoritative information with regard to the subject matter covered herein. It is sold with the clear understanding that the Publisher is not engaged in rendering legal or any other professional services. If legal or any other expert assistance is required, the services of a competent person should be sought. FROM A DECLARATION OF PARTICIPANTS JOINTLY ADOPTED BY A COMMITTEE OF THE AMERICAN BAR ASSOCIATION AND A COMMITTEE OF PUBLISHERS.

Additional color graphics may be available in the e-book version of this book.

Library of Congress Cataloging-in-Publication Data

ISBN: 978-1-62808-745-1

Library of Congress Control Number: 2013945713

Published by Nova Science Publishers, Inc. † New York

Contents

Preface

Bone is a dynamic tissue that undergoes continual adaptation during vertebrate life to attain and preserve skeletal size, shape, and structural integrity and to regulate mineral homeostasis. Bone homeostasis, which maintaines bone mass, is skillfully regulated through osteoclasts, osteoblasts and osteocytes, which are major cells in bone tissues. Many hormones and cytokines and immune systems implicate in the regulation of bone homeostasis.

Aging induces a reduction in bone mass. Bone mass is reduced by a decrease in osteoblastic bone formation and an increase in osteoclastic bone resorption. Osteoporosis with its accompanying decrease in bone mass is widely recognized as a major public health problem. The most dramatic expression of the disease is represented by fractures of the proximately femur, and the number of which increase as the population ages [1-3]. Moreover, bone loss has been shown to stimulate in various pathophysiologic states including inflammatary condition, obesity, diabetes, and cancer cell bone metastasis.

Malnutrition or undernutrition is often observed with increasing ages, and it appears to be more intense in patients with hip fracture than in the general aging population [4]. The deficiency in both micronutrients and macronutrients appears to be strongly implicated in the pathogenesis and consequences of hip fracture in the osteoporotic elderly. This may generate the concept that bone homeostasis is regulated through various nutritional and food factors.

There is growing evidence that nutritional and functional food factors have a role in the prevention of bone loss with increasing age [5]. Food life style may help to prevent bone loss with aging. Chemical compounds in food and plants, which regulate bone homeostasis, have been to be notice. Recent studies have been shown that nutritional and functional food factors, which are present in fruit and vegetables, stimulate osteoblastic bone formation and suppresse osteoclastic bone resorption in animal models and human subjects [5], thereby increasing bone mass. Supplemental intake of ingredients plays an important role in maintaining bone health and in the prevention of bone loss. This may provide a new tool in the treatment of osteoporosis, which is proposed as "biomedical osteoporosis treatment" in this book.

The author is engaged in the research fields concerning the elucidation of the role of nutritional and functional food factors in the regulation of bone homeostasis and in the prevention and treatment of osteoporosis since 1984. This book is writtened to be based on the topics which were generated in various biomedical systems in bone cells, animal models, and human subjects.

This book, which was entitled as "Biomedical Osteoporosis Treatment", has been composed in Chapter 1 to 14.

Chapter 1: This chapter introduces the outline of bone homeostasis and involvement of osteoporosis. Bone is a dynamic tissue that undergoes continual adaptation during vertebrate life to attain and preserve skeletal size, shape, and structural integrity and to regulate mineral homeostasis. Two processes, remodeling and modeling, underpin development and maintenance of the skeletal system. Bone modeling is responsible for growth and mechanically induced adaptation of bone and requires the processes of bone formation and bone removal (resorption). Bone remodeling is responsible for removal and repair of damaged bone to maintain integrity of the adult skeletal and mineral homeostasis. Bone homeostasis is regulated through various physiological systems and it is disturbed through various pathophysiological states which induce osteoporosis. This chapter describes a regulatory mechanism of bone homeostasis and an involvement in osteoporosis.

Chapter 2: Zinc plays a pivotal role as an essential nutritional factor in the growth of animals and human. Bone growth retardation is a common finding in various conditions associated with dietary zinc deficiency. Bone zinc content has been shown to decrease in aging, skeletal unloading and postmenopausal conditions, suggesting its role in bone disorder. Zinc has been demonstrated to have stimulatory effects on osteoblastic bone formation and mineralization due to stimulating cellular protein synthesis and the gene expression of the transcription factors runt-related transcription factor 2 (Runx 2) which is related to differentiation into osteoblastic cells. Moreover, zinc has been shown to inhibit osteoclastic bone resorption due to inhibiting osteoclast-like cell formation from bone marrow cells and stimulating apoptotic cell death of mature osteoclasts. Zinc has a suppressive effect on the receptor activator of nuclear factor (NF)-κB ligand (RANKL)-induced osteoclastogenesis. Interestingly, zinc transporter has been shown to express in osteoblastic cells and osteoclastic cells. Intake of dietary zinc causes an increase in bone mass. β-Alanyl-L-histidinato zinc and zinc asexamate, which are a new zinc compound, have been shown to have stimulatory effects on bone formation with more intensive than that of zinc sulfate. Oral administration of these zinc compounds has potent-restorative effects on bone loss under various pathophysiologic conditions including aging, skeletal unloading, aluminium bone toxicity, calcium- and vitamin D-deficiency, adjuvant arthritis, estrogen deficiency, diabetes, and fracture healing. Zinc compounds may be designed as new supplementation factor in the prevention and treatment of osteoporosis.

Chapter 3: Genistein is a functional food factor, which is largely contained in soybeans. Genistein has been shown to have a stimulatory effect on osteoblastic bone formation and a suppressive effect on osteoclastic bone resorption, thereby increasing bone mass. Genistein stimulates osteoblastogenesis and suppresses osteoclastogenesis. This factor has regulatory effects on protein synthesis and gene expression, which are related to bone formation in osteoblastic cells and bone resorption in osteoclastic cells. Oral administration of genistein has been shown to prevent on bone loss in ovariectomized rats, an animal model for osteoporosis, indicating a role in the prevention of osteoporosis. Moreover, the intake of dietary soybean genistein has been shown to have a restorative effect on osteoporosis in human subjects, suggesting a role in the treatment of bone loss.

Chapter 4: Both zinc and genistein are largely contained in soybeans. Combination of zinc and genistein has been found to have synergistic stimulatory effects on osteoblastic bone formation and synergistic suppressive effects on osteoclastic bone resorption, thereby increasing bone mass. These factors have effects on protein synthesis and gene expression, which are related to osteoblastic bone formation and osteoclastic bone resorption. Oral administration with the combination of zinc and genistein was found to have synergistic preventive effects on bone loss in ovariectomized rats, an animal model for osteoporosis, indicating a role in the treatment of osteoporosis. Moreover, supplemental intake of ingrediant with the combination of zinc and genistein has been shown to have potent effects on osteoporosis in human subjects. Combination of functional food factors may be potential tools in the prevention and treatment of osteoporosis.

Chapter 5: Vitamin K is known as a blood coagulative factor. There are three types of vitamin K: vitamin K_1 (phylloquinone), vitamin K_2 (menaquinone), and vitamin K_3 (menadione). Menaquinone-4 (MK-4), with four isoprene units, not only enhances mineralization but also increases amount of osteocalcin, which has a high affinity to calcium and/or hydroxyapataite, in human osteoblasts. MK-4 has been shown to inhibit bone resorption and inhibits bone loss in ovariectomized rats. Menaquinone-7 (MK-7) with seven isoprene units is very abundant in fermented soybean. Dietary vitamin K intake has beneficial effects on bone. MK-7 has a stimulatory effect on osteoblastic bone formation due to increasing protein synthesis including osteocalcin. Also, MK-7 has an inhibitory effect on osteoclastogenesis. Suppressive effects of MK-7 on osteoclasts may be partly mediated through the pathway of Ca^{2+}- and cyclic AMP-dependent signaling. The actions of MK-7 on osteoblasts and osteoclasts are accomplished by downregulating basal and cytokine-induced the nuclear factor kappa B (NF-κB) activation, by increasing IκB mRNA, in a γ-carboxylation–independent manner. Vitamin K_2 is a transcriptional regulator of bone-specific genes that act through steroid and xenobiotic receptors (SXRs) to promote expression of osteoblastic markers. The intake of dietary MK-7 has a preventive effect on bone loss caused by ovariectomy in rats *in vivo*. The intake of dietary MK-7 with reinforced natto (fermented soybean) can stimulate γ-carboxylation of osteocalcin in normal human subjects. Dietary MK-7 may be useful in the prevention and treatment of osteoporosis.

Chapter 6: Vitamin A (retinol, retinal and retinoic acid), which is formed from carotenoids in animal and human, has an anabolic effect on bone, and it is also known to have a detrimental effect on bone at high doses. Among various carotenoids (carotene and xanthophylls including β-cryptoxanthin, lutein, lycopene, β-carotene, astaxanthin and rutin), β-cryptoxanthin has been found to have a stimulatory effect on bone calcification *in vitro*.β-Cryptoxanthin is abundant in Satsuma mandarin orange (*Citrus unshiu* MARC.). β-Cryptoxanthin has stimulatory effects on osteoblastic bone formation and inhibitory effects on osteoclastic bone resorption *in vitro*, thereby increasing bone mass. β-Cryptoxanthin has effects on the gene expression of various proteins, which are related to osteoblastic bone formation and osteoclastic bone resororption *in vitro*. Oral administration of β-cryptoxanthin has been shown to have a preventive effect on bone loss in animal models for osteoporosis *in vivo*. The intake of β-cryptoxanthin-reinforced orange juice has been shown to have stimulatory effects on bone formation and suppressive effects on bone resorption in healthy human or postmenopausal women. Epidemiological studies suggest a potential role of β-cryptoxanthin as a sustainable nutritional approach to improving bone health of human subjects.

Chapter 7: Bioactive flavonoid *p*-hydroxycinnamic acid (HCA) is an intermediate-metabolic substance in plants and fruits and is synthesized from tyrosine. Among of cinnamic acid, HCA, ferulic acid, caffeic acid, or 3, 4-dimethoxycinnamic acid which are present in plants, HCA has been uniquely found to have a potent-anabolic effect on bone mineralization *in vitro*. HCA stimulates osteoblastic bone formation and suppresses osteoclastic bone resorption *in vitro*. Oral administration of HCA was found to have preventive effects on bone loss induced with ovarietomy and diabetic state. HCA may have effects in the prevention and treatment of osteoporosis.

Chapter 8: Flavonoid, a kind of polyphenol, possesses a fundmental chemical structure of flavone and displays yellow pigments, including flavone, isoflavon, flavonol, flavonon and quercetin, which are found in fruits, vegetables, leaves and grains. Flavonoid has a strong anti-oxidant effect. In recent years, flavonoid has been shown to have an effect on bone. Quercetin, a flavonol, is a plant-derived flavonoid. It is used as an ingredient in supplements, beverages or foods. Quercetin has been shown to have a stimulatory effect on osteoblastic bone formation and a suppressive effect on osteoclastic bone resorption. Quercetin suppresses NF-κB activation, which is mediated through TNF-α and RANKL in osteoblastogenesis and osteoclastogenesis. Oral administration of quercetin has been shown to have preventive and treatment effects on estrogen deficiency-induced bone loss in ovariectomized animals, a model of menopausal osteoporosis. Supplemental intake of dietary quercetin may have a role in the treatment of osteoporosis.

Chapter 9: Curcumin is a principal curcuminoid of the popular Indian spice turmeric, which is a member of the ginger family (*Zingiberaceae*). Curcumin may be useful for the prevention and treatment of several diseases. In both *in vitro* and animal studies, curcumin has been shown to have antitumor, antioxidant, antiarthritic, antiamyloid, anti-ischemic, and anti-inflammatory properties. As of 2008, clinical trials in humans were underway, studying the effect of curcumin on various diseases, including multiple myeloma, pancreatic cancer, myelodysplastic syndromes, colon, psoriasis, and Alzheimer's disease. Curcumin and its related compounds have been shown to regulate bone homeostasis *in vitro*. Curcumin has a stimulatory effect on osteoblastogenesis and a suppressive effect on osteoclastogenesis. Curcumin suppresses NF-κB activation, which is mediated through RANKL and TNF-α in osteoclastogenesis. Oral administration of curcumin has been shown to have restorative effects on menopausal-induced bone loss using animal models *in vivo*, suggesting a role in the prevention and treatment in osteoporosis. Moreover, UBS109, a novel carcumin analogue, has been found to have potent effects on the stimulation of osteoblastogenesis and suppression of osteoclastogenesis. An applicative usefulness in osteoporosis treatment may be expected.

Chapter 10: Consumption of green tea, a rich source of epigallocatechin-3-gallate (EGCG), is associated with increased bone mineral density, suggesting a role in the prevention of osteoporosis. EGCG has been demonstrated to have stimulatory effects on osteoblastogenesis and mineralization and suppressive effects on osteoclastogenesis and bone resorption *in vitro*. Supplementation of green tea extract and EGCG prevented bone loss induced in ovariectomized rats *in vivo*, supporting the view that dietary EGCG may be useful in the prevention and treatment of osteoporosis.

Chapter 11: Magnolia officinalis, a component of Asian herbal teas, has long been employed in traditional Japanese and Chinese medicine to treat numerous maladies. Honokiol, a biphenolic compound, is now considered to be one of the major active ingredients of *Magnolia* extract, and is under intense investigation for its anti-angiogenic, anti-inflammatory, antitumor and neuroprotective properties. Honokiol has been shown to have stimulatory effects on osteoblastogenesis and mineralization and suppressive effects on osteoclastogenesis *in vitro*. The adiministration of honokiol has been demonstrated to suppress prostate cancer cell bone metastasis in mice *in vivo*, suggesting that honokiol has an inhibitory effect on cancer cell-induced osteolysis. In addition, honokiol may be expected to have effects in the prevention and treatment of osteoporosis.

Chapter 12: Among marine algae of *Undaria pinnatifida, Sargassum horneri, Eisenia bicyclis, Cryptonemia scmitziana, Gelidium amansii,* and *Ulva pertusa* Kjellman, which are used as food in East Asian, *Sargassum horneri (S. horneri)* is found to have a unique anabolic effect on bone components. *S. horneri* extract had stimulatory effects on osteoblastic bone formation and inhibitory effects on osteoclastic bone resorption *in vitro*, thereby increasing bone mass. The active component is found to be less than molecular weight 3000 in the extract. The intake of *S. horneri* extract caused a preventive effect on bone loss in animal models for osteoporosis and in healthy human. *S. horneri* extract may be usefull as an osteogenic factor in the prevention of osteoporosis in human subjects.

Chapter 13: Among various food and plants (including shiitake, loquat leaf, cherry leaf, gabaron tea, green tea, muskmelon, tomato, blueberry, and wasabi leafstalk), the active component, which stimulates bone mineralization in mouse bone tissues *in vitro,* is found to be present in the leafstalk of wasabi (*Wasabi japanica* MATSUM). The material with a low molecular weight of 158 may be the active component in wasabi leafstalk which stimulates bone mineralization. Supplemental intake of wasabi leafstalk components may have effects on the prevention and treatment of osteoporosis.

Chapter 14: Among of royal jelly, propolis and bee pollen, the water soluble extract obtained from bee pollen *Cistus ladaniferus* has been found to have a direct anabolic effect on bone tissues *in vitro*. Bee pollen extract has stimulatory effects on osteoblastic bone formation and suppressive effects on osteoclastogenesis and bone resorption *in vitro*. Supplemental intake of bee pollen extract prevented bone loss in overiectomized and streptozotocin-induced diabetic rats *in vivo*. Supplemental intake of bee pollen extract may play a role in the prevention and treatment of osteoporosis.

As described above, functional food factors play an important role in the regulation of bone homeostasis and in the prevention and treatment of osteoporosis in various pathophysiological states. Analogues, which are synthesized with the origination of bioactive chemicals in food factors, may be developed as novel drugs that reveal potent-osteogenic effects for the treatment of osteolysis in various diseases including osteoporosis, cancer cell bone metastasis, and bone fracture.

The author expects that this book will be focused with much interestings on many scientists in the fields of biomedical research. In addition, the author believes that the supplemental intake of biomedical food ingredients may play a role in the prevention and treatment of osteoporosis and that will be contributed to health care of people.

Finally, the author thanks Nova Science Publishers, Inc., which was given me the opportunity of publication of this book.

July, 2013

Masayoshi Yamaguchi, PhD, IOM, FAOE, DDG, DG
E-mail: yamamasa1155@yahoo.co.jp

Chapter 1

Bone Homeostasis and Osteoporosis

Bone is a dynamic tissue that undergoes continual adaptation during vertebrate life to attain and preserve skeletal size, shape, and structural integrity and to regulate mineral homeostasis. Two processes, remodeling and modeling, underpin development and maintenance of the skeletal system. Bone modeling is responsible for growth and mechanically induced adaptation of bone and requires that the processes of bone formation and bone removal (resorption), although globally coordinated, occur independently at distinct anatomical locations. Bone remodeling is responsible for removal and repair of damaged bone to maintain integrity of the adult skeletal and mineral homeostasis. This tightly coordinated event requires the synchronized activities of multiple cellular participates to ensure that bone resorption and formation occur sequentially at the same anatomical location to preserve bone mass.

Regulation of Bone Homeostasis

Bone contains over 98% of total body calcium. Bone homeostasis is regulated with the functions of osteoblasts and osteoclasts, which are major cells in bone tissue [6-9]. Osteoblasts, which are differentiated from bone marrow messenchymal stem cells, stimulate bone formation and calcification, while osteoclasts, which develop from hematopoietic progenitors, promote bone resorption. In the physiologic process of bone turnover, a resorptive stimulus firstly triggers recruitment of osteoclasts to a site on the bone surface. Osteoclasts, which develop from hematopoietic progenitors, are recruited to the site and excavate the calcified matrix. After resorbed lacunar pit is filled with new osteoid, osteoblasts become flatter and less active, with the final newly remodeled bone surface lined by flat lining cells. Remodeling of cancellous bone begins with the retraction of lining cells that cover the bone surface. Then, the cavity is refilled by osteoblasts via a process that occurs in three distinct phases: initiation, progression and termination. During the initiation phase, a team of osteoblasts arising from local mesenchymal stem cells assembles at the bottom of the cavity and bone formation begins.

As bone formation progresses, some osteoblasts are entombed within the matrix as osteocytes but the majority dies by apoptosis. Bone formation terminates when the cavity has been refilled, at which time the few osteoblasts that remain become the flat lining cells that cover the quiescent surfaces of bone. Once formed, few osteocytes die. Their viability is likely maintained by physiological levels of mechanical stimulation. When mechanical forces are reduced for example in weightlessness, osteocytes die by apoptosis. This event appears to act as a beacon for osteoclast recruitment and generation of a new basic multicellular unit, which in turn replaces the old bone containing dead osteocytes with new bone containing viable osteocytes.

The process of bone remodeling is regulated with respect to the interactions along the remodeling sequence by systemic influences (hormones and cytokines), the stress action on trabecular and cortical systems with physical activity and weight bearing, various growth factors produced from the bone cells which act locally on the cells, or other factors that come from nearby cells present in the marrow tissues. The physiological bone remodeling is a highly coordinated process responsible for bone resorption and formation and is necessary to repair damaged bone and to maintain mineral homeostasis [10]. In addition to traditional bone cells (osteoclasts, osteoblasts, and osteocytes) which are necessary for bone remodeling, several immune cells have also been implicated in bone disease.

Bone acts as major storage site for growth factors, which are produced by osteoblasts, diffuse into newly deposited osteoid and are stored in the bone matrix including isulin-like growth factors (IGF-I and -II), transforming growth factor-β1 (TGF-β1), platelet-derived growth factor (PDGF), or bone morphologic proteins (BMPs) [11, 12]. These bone-derived factors, which can be liberated during subsequent periods of bone resorption, act in an autocrine, paracrine, or delayed paracrine fashion in the local microenvironment of the bone surface. The process of bone remodeling to make bone is unique among organs and tissues, and it is complexity with respect to interactions along the remodeling sequence by systemic influences (hormones including parathyroid hormone, calcitonin, 1, 25-dihydroxyvitamin D_3, and estrogen and cytokines including tumor necrosis factor-α), stress action on the trabecular and cortical systems, growth factors and cytokines produced by bone cells which act locally on their own cell types and on the other bone cell types, or factors that come from nearby cells present in the bone marrow tissues. The regulatory process of bone homeostasis is summarized in Figure 1.

There is growing evidence that zinc finger transcription factors, which are zinc-binding protein, play an important role in the differentiation of osteoblastic cells and osteoclastic cells. Zinc transporter has been shown to locate in osteoblastic cells [13] and osteoclastic cells [14]. Zinc transporter may be important role in the uptake, intracellular sequestration or efflux of zinc. A novel zinc finger-containing transcription factor, called Osterix (Osx), has been found in osteoblastic cells [15]. Osx is specifically expressed in all developing bones. Osx is required for osteoblast differentiation and bone formation, and it acts downstream of Runx2/Cbfa1 [15]. Cas-interacting zinc finger protein (CIZ) has been found to be a novel type inhibitor of bone morphogenetic protein (BMP)/Smad signaling in modulation of BMP2-induced osteoblastic cell differentiation [16]. Moreover, Schnurri-3 (Shn3), a mammalian homolog of the Drosophila zinc finger adapter protein Shn, is an essential regulator of adult bone formation [17]. Runx2-mediated extracellular matrix mineralization is antagonized, revealing an essential role for Shn3 as a central regulator of postnatal bone mass. A novel TIZ (TRAF6-inhibitory zinc finger protein) has been shown to inhibit osteoclastogenesis and function of tumor necrosis factor receptor-associated factor 6 [18]. TIZ may play a regulatory role during osteoclast differentiation by modulating TRAF6 signaling activity. Whether nutritional zinc state may affect on the function of zinc finger proteins has been poorly understood. Thus, zinc is essentially related to the functions of various zinc-proteins, which participate in cellular regulation of bone homeostasis.

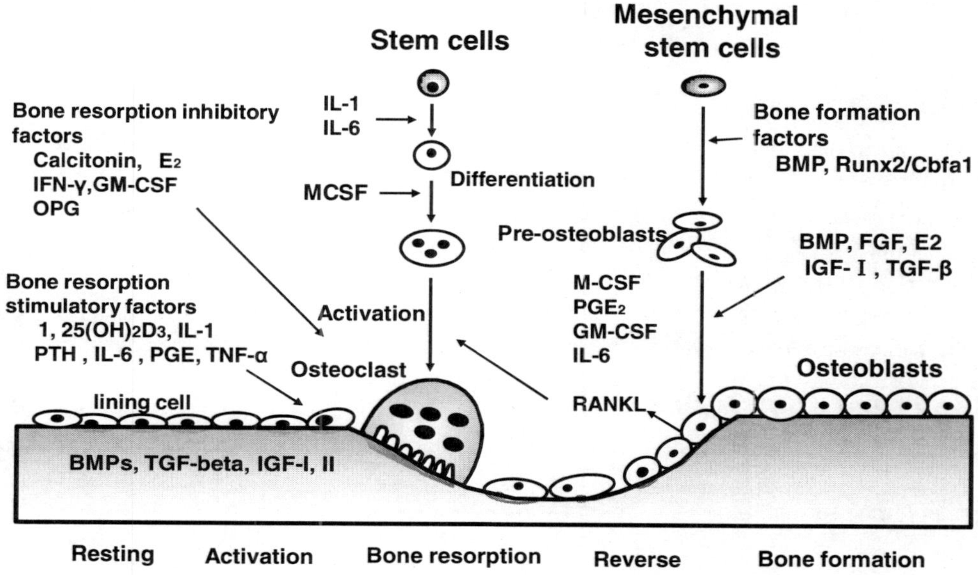

Figure 1. Regulatory mechanism of bone remodeling. Bone metabolism is regulated by osteoclasts and osteoblasts. Osteoclasts, which stimulate bone resorption, are generated from stem cells by interleukin-1 (IL-1), IL-6, M-CSF, and other factors. Osteoclastogenesis is mediated through RANKL produced from osteoblasts by various bone resorption-stimulating factors. Osteoblasts, which stimulate bone formation and mineralization, are differentiated from mesenchymal stem cells by various bone formation factors. After bone formation and mineralization, osteoblasts are changed to osteocytes in bone matrix. Bone growth factors [transforming growth factor-beta (TGF- β), bone morphogenetic proteins (BMPs), and insulin-like growth factor-I and –II (IGF-I and IGF-II)], which are produced by osteoblasts, are accumulated in bone matrix. These factors are released by bone resorption into the bone surface and contribute bone formation.

Disorder of Bone Homeostasis Induces Osteoporosis

As described above, bone homeostasis is skillfully regulated through osteoclasts and osteoblasts. Bone mass with increasing ages is reduced by decrease in osteoblactic bone formation and increase in osteoclastic bone resorption, thereby inducing osteoporosis. Osteoporosis, which is characterized by reduced bone strength and an increased risk for low-trauma fractures, increases dramatically with age. About 40% of women in developed countries will experience an osteoporosis-related fracture in the course of their lifetime, with men experiencing approximately one-third to one-half the risk of women [19, 20]. Thus, osteoporosis is a major cause of increased morbidity and mortality affecting the aging population. The most dramatic expression of osteoporosis is represented by fractures of the proximal femur for which the number increases as the population ages.

Bone mass is dramatically reduced after menopause, which depresses the secretion of ovarian hormone (estrogen) in women [3]. The deficiency of estrogen advances osteoclastic bone resorption. This is very important as a primary osteoporosis. Postmenopausal osteoporosis, a consequence of ovarian hormone deficiency, is the archetypal osteoporotic condition in women after menopause and leads to bone destruction through complex and diverse metabolic and biochemical changes.

In addition, osteoporosis has been shown to induce after diabetes (type I and II), obesity, inflammatory disease, and various pathophysiological states. In recent years, diabetic osteoporosis is noticed. Diabetes is frequent in the elderly, and therefore frequently coexists with osteoporosis [20, 21]. Furthermore, there has also been a global increase in the prevalence of obesity, with obesity-related diabetes currently affecting over 366 million adults worldwide and projections that this will reach 552 million by 2030 [22]. Type 1 diabete, and more recently type 2 diabete, has been associated with increased fracture risk. High glucose levels in type 2 diabete lead to accumulation of advanced glycosylation end-products (AGEs) in the organic bone matrix by a process known as nonenzymatic glycation [20]. There is evidence suggesting that AGEs interfere with normal osteoblast development, function and attachement to the collagen matrix [20]. Increased AGEs may weaken bone by decreasing bone formation.

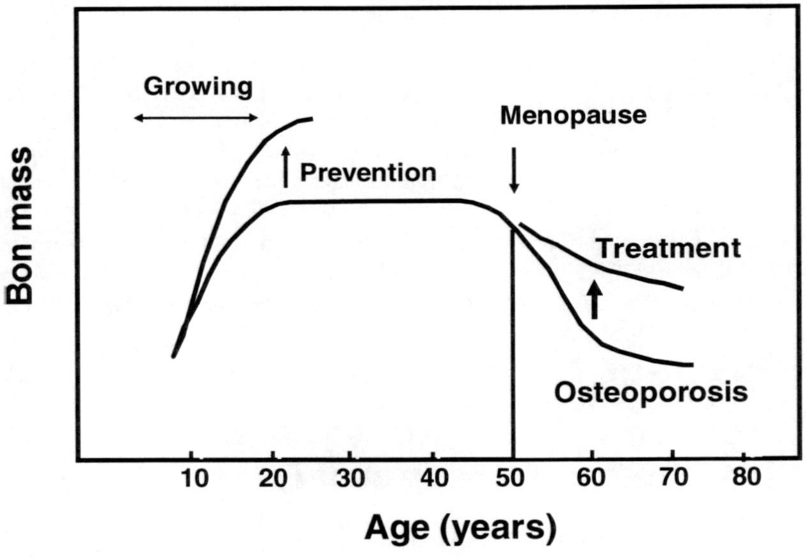

Figure 2. Change in bone mass with increasing age. Bone mass increases with growing and reaches to peak in the range of age between twenty and twenty-five years. Then, bone mass is gradually decreased with aging. In menopausal women, bone mass dramatically decreases and this bone loss leads to osteoporosis. Estrogen deficiency with menopause stimulates osteoblastic bone resorption and suppresses osteoblastic bone formation, thereby inducing bone mass. In addition, bone mass is reduced in other pathophysiological states including hyperlipidemia, obesity, diabetes, inflammation, and cancer bone metastasis. It is important to prevent and to treat decrease in bone mass with pathophysilogic states.

In Western societies, mean body weight has increased dramatically in older people, and a similar trend exists in Asia. Yet insufficient attention has been directed to the problem of osteoporotic fractures in the overwight and obese [23]. Osteoporotic fractures occur in overweight or obese people, and obese men may be particularly susceptible [23]. The National Health and Nutrition Examination Survey have reported that 63% of osteoporotic patients have hyperlipidemia [24]. Epidemiological studies reveal an inverse relationship between serum cholesterol levels and bone mineral content and density [25], independent of age and body mass index. Diet-induced hyperlipidemia is also associated with a reduction in bone mineral content and density in animals [26]. Hyperlipidemia induces secondary hyperparathyroidism and impairs bone regeneration and mechanical strength [27].

The change in bone mass with increasing age is shown in Figure 2. There is growing evidence that many functional food factors (biomedical food factors) regulate bone homeostasis and that have beneficial effects in the prevention and treatment of osteoporosis, which is induced in various pathophysiological states.

Chapter 2

Role of Nutritional Zinc in Bone Homeostasis: Osteoporosis Treatment with Zinc Compound

Zinc, a nutritional trace element, is essential for the growth of human and animals [28-30]. Zinc is required for the growth, development, and maintenance of healthy bones. Bone growth retardation is a common finding in various conditions associated with zinc deficiency [31-35]. In Iranian schoolboys at year 1961, zinc supplementation was firstly found to restore both skeletal growth and maturation [36]. Zinc deficiency is associated with many kinds of skeletal abnormalities in fetal and postnatal development. Zinc may play a physiologically important role in bone homeostasis.

Skeleton contains a large proportion of the total body burden of zinc [37]. Bone zinc has been shown to be concentrated in the layer of osteoid prior to calcification [38]. Zinc can be mobilized by conditions such as calcium deficiency in the pregnant rats [39]. Early mobilization of maternal bone provided sufficient zinc prevents fetal malformation, and most fetal zinc is derived from maternal muscle mobilized later in the calcium-deficient pregnancy [40].

Bone appears to act as a zinc sink. Zinc is released during skeletal breakdown, and it is mostly reincorporated into the skeleton [41, 42]. In human, the vertebral calcium/zinc is inversely related to age, suggesting that skeletal zinc is conserved more than calcium in later life [43]. Zinc also occurs in the mineral component of bone, probably in hydroxyapatite [44]; it may be complex with fluoride; and both zinc and the zinc-fluoride complex may improve the crystallinity of apatite.

Osteoporotic patients have been shown to have lower levels of skeletal zinc than control [45]. In postmenopausal women, urinary zinc has been suggested as a marker of bone resorption, since women with osteoporosis excrete over than 800 μg zinc/g creatinine in urine [46]. The supplements of trace minerals with or without calcium in postmenopausal women have been shown to have beneficial effects on bone density [46].

Zinc may play a physiologically important role in bone. The mechanism of action of zinc on osteoblastic and osteoclastic cells that regulate bone homeostasis, however, has been poorly defined. In recent years, there is growing evidence that zinc has an important role in the regulation of bone homeostasis. Zinc has been demonstrated to stimulate osteoblastic bone formation and to inhibit osteoclastic bone resorption, thereby increasing bone mass. Supplementation of nutritional zinc has been shown to have preventive and therapeutic effects on bone loss that is induced in various bone disorders.

This chapter has been written to outline the recent advances concerning the role of zinc in regulation of bone homeostasis and in the prevention and therapy of osteoporosis.

Nutritional Zinc Has Anabolic Effects on Bone

Zinc has anabolic effects on bone metabolism *in vivo* and *in vitro*. Oral administration of zinc sulfate (5 and 10 mg Zn/kg body weight) for 3 days produced dose-dependent increases in the contents of zinc, deoxyribonucleic acid (DNA), collagen and calcium, and the activity of alkaline phosphatase in the femoral diaphysis (cortical bone) of weanling rats [47]. Alkaline phosphatase is related to bone mineralization in osteoblasts [48]. Collagen is a main bone matrix protein which is produced in osteoblasts [48]. DNA content in bone tissues is a marker of the number of bone cells, including osteoblasts, osetoclasts, and osteocytes [49]. Zinc accumulated in the bone tissues may firstly cause the activation of alkaline phosphatase and the stimulation of collagen synthesis in osteoblasts, which are involved in bone mineralization and calcification.

The anbolic effects of metal on bone were not seen in other essential trace metals [50-52]. Oral administration of chromium (III), cobalt, copper, manganese, nickel, and selenium (15.3 μmol as metal/kg) for 3 days caused a significant increase in the diaphyseal alkaline phosphatase activity and DNA content, while the doses of 153 μmol/kg clearly decreased the enzyme activity. The dose of germanium (306 μmol /kg) caused a significant decrease in the diaphyseal alkaline phosphatase activity and DNA content. Supplememtation with copper in adequate copper nutrition does not have anabolic effects on bone components [52]. Oral administration of zinc with the dose of 3,060 μmol /kg produced increases in both alkaline phosphatase activity and DNA content in the diaphyseal tissues. Zinc has the lowest toxicity for bone metabolism as compared with other trace metals.

Zinc has stimulatory effects on bone formation in tissue culture system *in vitro*. Calvaria were removed from weanling rats and cultured for a period up to 96 hours in Dulbecco's Modified Eagle Medium [53]. Zinc uptake by bone tissues was significantly increased after culture with zinc. Bone calcium content was significantly increased in the presence of 10^{-4} M zinc. The physiological zinc concentration in the serum was in the range of 10^{-4} to 4 x10^{-4} M. Bone alkaline phosphatase and ATPase activities were increased in the presence of zinc (10^{-6} to 10^{-3} M), whereas it did not change significantly the activities of pyrophosphatase, acid phosphatase, and β-N-acetylglucosaminidase. Bone collagen content was raised in the presence of zinc. The effects of zinc in increasing bone alkaline phosphatase activity and collagen content have been shown to prevent after the administration of an inhibitor of protein synthesis, suggesting that bone protein synthesis is a necessary component of this response.

The first steps in the biosynthesis of protein involve the enzymatic activation of amino acids with adenosine triphosphate, followed by the transfer of amino acids to amino acid-specific ribonucleic acids (RNA). The presence of zinc in the culture medium has been found to induce a significant increase in the incoporation of [^{3}H]-leucine into acid-insoluble residues of bone tissue [54]. The activity of [^{3}H] leucyl-tRNA synthetase in the 105,000 *g* supernatant fraction (cytosol) of the bone homogenate was increased about twofold after culture with zinc [55]. Zinc has a direct stimulatory effect on protein synthesis at the translational level in bone cells *in vitro*.

Endogenous zinc in the bone tissues has also been shown to play an essential role on bone protein synthesis in the culture [55]. When the calvaria were cultured for 24 hours in a medium containing dipicolinate (10^{-6} to 10^{-3} M), a chelator of zinc, bone zinc content was decreased after culture with dipicolinate [55]. In this case, bone alkaline phoshatase activity was decreased by about 40% of untreated bone enzyme activity. Decreased alkaline phosphatase activity was markedly increased in the presence of 10^{-4} M zinc (about 2.5-fold of control value). The effect of zinc was completely blocked after culture with protein synthesis inhibitor. Thus, bone endogenous zinc plays a role in the stimulation of protein synthesis at the translational process in bone cells. Zinc has been shown to increase many constitutive proteins in bone tissues *in vitro* [56].

Zinc has been shown to enhance anabolic effects of vitamin D_3 on bone components in the femur of weanling rats *in vivo* [57]. The administration of vitamin D_3 (10 μg/kg) or zinc (10 mg Zn/kg) produced a significant increase in bone alkaline phosphatase activity and DNA content. The increase in alkaline phosphatase activity was additionally enhanced by the simultaneous administration of vitamin D_3 and zinc. The increase in bone DNA content was markedly (about fourfold) enhanced by both treatments. These increases were prevented after the administration of cycloheximide, an inhibitor of protein synthesis [58, 59]. The effects of 1, 25-dihydroxyvitamin D_3 (0.5 and 1.5 μg/kg) in increasing bone alkaline phosphatase activity and DNA content were synergistically enhanced after the simultaneous treatment with zinc [59]. The receptors for 1, 25-dihydroxyvitamin D_3 [1, $25(OH)_2D_3$] are shown to have two zinc fingers at the sit of interaction with DNA [60]. Zinc may potentiate the interaction of 1, $25(OH)_2D_3$-receptor with DNA at that site. These findings suggest that combination of vitamin D_3 and zinc has synergistic effects on the stimulation of bone growth and mineralization in rats *in vivo*.

Zinc has also been shown to modulate hormonal effects on bone formation and calcification in bone tissue culture *in vitro*. The presence of 1, $25(OH)_2D_3$ produced a significant increase in alkaline phosphatase activity, DNA and calcium contents in tissue culture with rat calvaria [61]. The anabolic effects of estrogen (17β-estradiol) on bone components in tissue culture were significantly enhanced after culture with zinc sulfate [62]. Such an effect was abolished with cycloheximide. Zinc modulates anabolic effects of 1, $25(OH)_2D_3$ or estrogen on bone metabolism *in vitro*. Zinc has been reported to increase the activity of 1, $25(OH)_2D_3$-dependent promoters in osteoblastic cells [63].

Zinc Stimulates Osteoblastic Bone Formation

The cellular mechanism of zinc action in stimulating bone formation has been demonstrated in osteobalstic MC3T3-E1 cells. The proliferation of osteoblastic cells was stimulated after culture with zinc compound (zinc sulfate or zinc-chelating dipeptide) with or without fetal bovine serum [64]. Culture with zinc increased DNA content in the cells. Zinc-induced increases in cell proliferation and DNA content were prevented after culture with cycloheximide. The effect of zinc in stimulating cell proliferation may be mediated through protein synthesis [64]. Zinc has been shown to stimulate cell differentiation of osteoblastic cells [65]. Culture with zinc (10^{-7} to 10^{-5} M) produced remarkable increases in alkaline phosphatase activity and protein concentration in osteoblastic cells. These increases were also seen with prolonged culture (12-21 days). The effect of zinc was completely abolished after culture with cycloheximide.

The protein components in osteoblastic MC3T3-E1 cells cultured with zinc have been characterized [66]. The homogenate of cells was analyzed with SDS-polyacrylamide gel electrophoresis. Culture with zinc caused an appreciable increase in many protein components in the cells. Especially, the 66 kilo Dalton (kDa) and 44 kDa proteins, which are the major components from control cells, were clearly found to increase in the presence of zinc compound. Moreover, the concentrations of osteocalcin, IGF-I, or TGF-β1 in the culture medium secreted from osteoblastic cells were markedly increased after culture with zinc. Zinc has been found to increase the production of bone growth factors and bone matrix protein, which are involved in the stimulation of bone formation and mineralization in osteoblastic cells [66].

The effect of IGF-I in increasing protein concentration, DNA content and cell number in the cells was markedly enhanced in the presence of zinc [67]. The cellular alkaline phosphatase activity was synergistically increased in the presence of both IGF-I and zinc. Such an effect was not seen after culture with both insulin and zinc. The enhancement of IGF-I's anabolic effect after culture with zinc has been shown to mediate through signaling pathway of protein kinase C and protein phosphatase in osteoblastic cells.

Culture with zinc sulfate has also been shown to increase protein tyrosine phosphatase activity in the cells [68]. The effect of IGF-I in increasing the enzyme activity was enhanced after culture with zinc [68]. Such an effect was not seen with parathyroid hormone. Zinc modulates anabolic effects of IGF-I on protein tyrosine phosphatase activity and cell proliferation. Likewise, the effect of estrogen on the proliferation of osteoblastic cells has also been enhanced after culture with zinc compound.

The clarification of a molecular mechanism by which zinc stimulates bone protein synthesis has been attempted. Aminoacyl-tRNA synthetase is an enzyme that synthesizes aminoacyl-tRNA. Zinc has been found to activate [^{3}H]-leucyl-tRNA synthetase in the homogenate of osteoblastic cells [69].

Zinc has also been demonstrated to stimulate DNA synthesis in the homogenate of osteoblastic cells *in vitro* [70]. Culture with zinc compound clearly stimulated DNA synthesis in the homogenate of osteoblastic cells, when it was estimated with the incorporation of [^{3}H] deoxythimidine 5'-triphosphate into the DNA in the homogenate. The effect of zinc was completely abolished after culture with cycloheximide, suggesting that the action of zinc is based on newly synthesized protein components. The effect of zinc in stimulating DNA synthesis may mainly result from protein synthesis. Also, it is possible that zinc has an effect on the process of DNA synthesis that is involved in the direct activation of DNA polymerase that is a zinc enzyme.

Zinc has been shown to stimulate the expression of transcription factors runt-related transcription factor 2 (Runx2) mRNA, a transcription factor, which is related to the differentiation to pre-osteoblastic cells [71].

As mentioned above, the mechanism of zinc action in stimulating osteoblastic bone formation and mineralization has been summarized in Figure 3. Zinc stimulates cell proliferation, cell differentiation, and mineralization in osteoblasts, thereby promoting bone formation. The molecular mechanism of zinc action may be to stimulate gene expression of various proteins including Runx2/Cbfa 1 (Core binding factor alpha1), type I collagen, alkaline phosphatase and osteocalcin in the cells. Also, zinc increases production of IGF-I and TGF-β1 in the cells. Moreover, zinc enhances protein synthesis due to activating aminoacyl-tRNA synthetase, a rate-limiting enzyme at translational process, in osteoblastic cells. Thus, zinc has a potent stimulatory effect on osteoblasitc bone formation.

Interestingly, the effects of IGF-I or estrogen on cell proliferation have been shown to enhance by zinc. The molecular mechanism of zinc action on cell nuclear events remains to be elucidated.

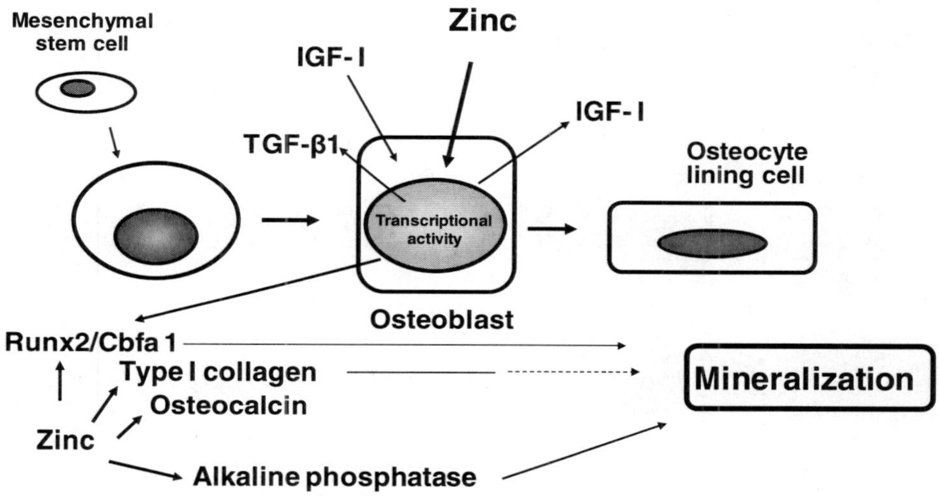

Figure 3. Cellular mechanism by which zinc stimulates osteoblastogenesis and mineralization. Zinc activates aminoacyl t-RNA synthetase at translational process and stimulates the gene expression of proteins, which are involved in osteoblastic bone formation and mineralization. Zinc stimulates differentiation and proliferation of preosteoblastic cells and enhances mineralization.

Zinc Suppresses Osteoclastic Bone Resorption

Zinc has suppressive effects on bone resorption [72]. Calvaria from weanling rats were cultured for periods of up to 48 hours in a medium containing various bone-resorbing factors [parathytoid hormone (PTH), prostaglandin E_2 (PGE_2), interleukin-1α (IL-1α), and lipopolysacharide]. These factors caused a significant decrease in bone calcium content. The decrease in bone calcium content was completely inhibited after culture with zinc compound [73]. Also, zinc compound completely inhibited PTH- or IL-1α-induced increases in medium glucose consumpion and lactic acid production by bone tissues [72]. The suppressive effects of zinc compound on bone resorption were not seen after culture with dipicolinate, a chelator of zinc. Thus, zinc has been shown to have suppressive effects on bone resorption in tissue culture system *in vitro*.

PGE_2 is secreted from osteoblasts. PTH or IL-1α caused a remarkable elevation of PGE_2 production in osteoblasts *in vitro* [73]. Culture with zinc compound did not have an effect on PGE_2 production in osteoblasts [73], indicating that the effect of zinc may not mediated through the suppression of PGE_2 production in osteoblasts.

Bone-resorbing cells, osteoclasts, are formed by differentiation of bone marrow cells. Zinc has an inhibitory effect on osteoclast-like cell formation in mouse marrow culture *in vitro* [74]. The bone marrow cells were cultured for 7 days in a medium containing bone-resorbing agent. Osteoclast-like cell formation was estimated staining for tartrate-resistant acid phosphatase (TRACP), a marker enzyme of osteoclasts. The presence of 1, 25-dihydroxyvitamin D_3, PTH, IL-1α, or PGE_2 induced a remarkable increase in osteoclast-like multinucleated cells. These increases were inhibited after culture with zinc (10^{-8} to 10^{-6} M). Suppressive effects of zinc compound were equal in comparison with the effect of other anti-bone resorbing agents (calcitonin, 17β-estradiol, or acetazolamide) on osteoclast-like cell formation in mouse marrow culture. When osteoclast isolated from rat femoral-diaphyseal tissues were cultured for 24 hours in the presence of zinc, the metal did not have effects on lysosomal enzyme activity (acid phosphatase or β-glucuronidase) in the cells [75]. Culture with zinc caused apoptotic cell death of mature osteoclast-like cells isolated in rat femoral tissues [75]. Zinc has been shown to have suppressive effects on osteoclastogenesis and osteoclastic cell death, which are generated with differentiation of bone marrow cells.

The mechanism of zinc action in inhibiting PTH-induced osteoclast-like cell formation in mouse marrow culture system *in vitro* has been shown [76]. The effect of zinc in inhibiting PTH-induced osteoclast-like cell formation was clearly seen in the presence or absence of theophylline. However, zinc did not inhibit a stimulatory effect of dibutyryl cyclic AMP on osteoclast-like cell formation. The stimulatory effects of PTH on osteoclast-like cell formation were clearly weakened (about 50%) in the presence of EGTA or dibucaine, a regulatory factor of intracellular Ca^{2+} signaling. Phorbol 12-myristate 13-acetate (PMA), a protein kinase C activator, stimulated osteoclast-like cell formation. Such an effect was suppressed after culture with zinc. However, suppressive effects of zinc were not seen in the presence of both PTH and PMA. These findings support the view that zinc suppresses PTH-stimulated osteoclast-like cell formation mediated through the Ca^{2+}-dependent activation of protein kinase C.

The receptor activator of NF-κB ligand (RANKL) plays a pivotal role in the development of osteoclasts from pre-osteoclasts [77, 78]. RANKL is secreted from osteoblasts. RANKL is a member of the tumor necrosis factor (TNF) superfamily, which was originally identified as T-cell-derived immunomodulatory cytokines [79]. RANKL is expressed in activated T cells and promotes the survival of dendritic cells by binding to its receptor RANK. RANKL/RANK pathway is essential for osteoclast differentiation [77, 78]. RANKL is expressed in osteoblastic cells and bone marrow stromal cells in response to osteotropic factors. The combined treatment of hematopoietic cells with macrophage-colony stimulating factor (M-CSF) and soluble from of RANKL (sRANKL) induces osteoclast differentiation *in vitro* [80]. The effect of RANKL was completely abrogated after addition of a natural antagonist of RANKL, osteoprotegerin (OPG) [81], which is produced in osteoblastic cells. TNF receptor-associated factor (TRAF) family proteins are adaptor molecules that mediate intracellular signaling of various cytokine receptors including the TNF receptor superfamily and Toll/interleukin receptor (IL-1R) family [82]. TRAF6 binds to the membrane-proximal region of RANK and IL-1R-associated kinase, and is critically involved in intracellular signal transduction including NF-κB and mitogen-activated protein kinase (MAPK) activation.

Zinc has been shown to have suppressive effects on RANKL-induced osteoclast-like cell formation in mouse marrow culture in the presence of M-CSF [83]. Zinc also inhibited TNF-α-induced osteoclastogenesis [83]. TNF-α is an autocrine factor in osteoclasts, promoting their differentiation, and mediates, at least in part, RANKL's induction of osteoclastogenesis [84]. The suppressive effects of zinc on osteoclastogenesis may be partly involved in the depressive effects on RANKL stimulation. In addition, zinc may inhibit signaling pathway that is related to RANKL stimulation in pre-osteoclasts.

The effect of zinc in inhibiting RANKL-induced osteoclastogenesis has been shown to abolish after culture with inhibitors of protein synthesis or transcription activity in mouse marrow cultures [83]. This finding suggests that the inhibitory effects of zinc on osteoclastogenesis are partly resulted from newly synthesized protein components that are involved in gene expression in mouse marrow culture.

Culture with zinc has been shown to have stimulatory effects on the expression of OPG mRNA in osteoblastic cells [71]. It is speculated that zinc stimulates the expression of RANKL inhibitor (including OPG) in osteoblasts, and that the metal induces a factor which suppresses osteoclast development in pre-osteoclasts.

As mentioned above, the cellular and molecular mechanism by which zinc inhibits osteoclastogenesis has been summarized in Figure 4.

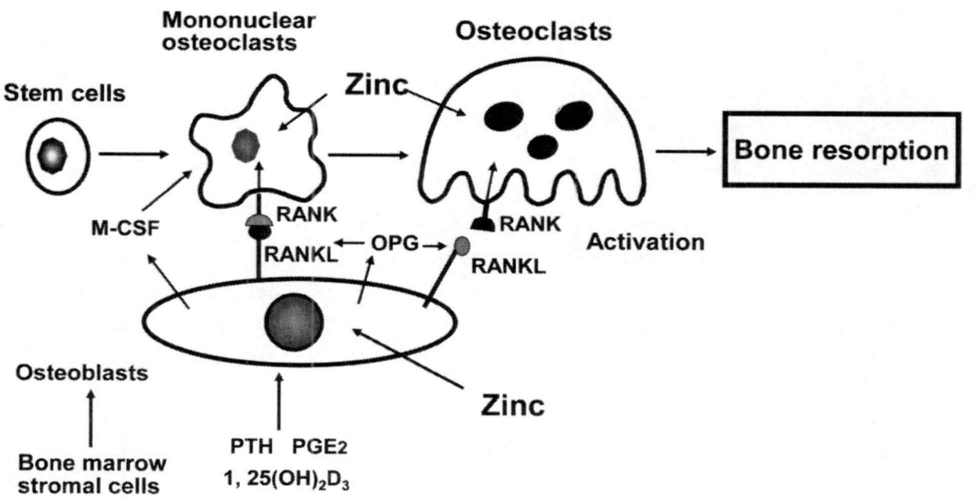

Figure 4. Cellular mechanism by which zinc inhibits osteoclastic bone resorption. Zinc suppresses osteoclast-like cell formation that is induced by various bone-resorbing factors in bone marrow culture at the later stage of osteoclastogenesis. This suppressive effect is based on the inhibition of RANKL action by zinc in pre-osteoclasts. Zinc also stimulates gene expression of OPG that can inhibit the binding of RANKL to RANK receptors in the cells. Zinc has a suppressive effect on acid production in osteoclastic cells.

Role of Zinc in Bone Growth

Zinc is an essential element for the growth of human and animals. Nutritional zinc is required for the growth, development and maintenance of healthy bones. Bone growth retardation is a common finding in various conditions associated with zinc deficiency [31-35]. In fact, zinc has been demonstrated to stimulate bone growth in newborn rats supplied with lactation by maternal rats [85]. Newborn rats were killed between 1 and 35 days after birth. Increasing age caused a significant increase in zinc and calcium contents and alkaline phosphatase activity in the femoral-diaphyseal and -metaphyseal tissues. Oral administration of zinc sulfate (20 mg Zn/kg body weight) with four times at 24-hour intervals to maternal rats from 1 day after birth induced a significant increase in zinc, alkaline phosphatase activity, DNA and calcium contents in the femoral-diaphyseal and -metaphyseal tissues of newborn rats compared with those at 7 or 14 days old [85], indicating that the increase in bone components results from lactation with zinc-containing milk of maternal rats. Zinc plays a physiological role in development of bone growth in newborn rats [85].

Endogenous zinc may be important in protein synthesis in the femoral-diaphyseal and -metaphyseal tissues of newborn rats [86]. Bone tissues were obtained at 1, 7, 14, 21, and 28 days after birth. Many protein molecules were found to be present in the bone tissues using SDS-polyacrylamide gel electrophoresis analysis. Bone protein synthesis activity was enhanced with increasing age, and reached a plateau 21 days after birth. Protein synthesis in the diaphyseal and metaphyseal tissues obtained from 7- or 14-day-old rats was significantly decreased after culture with a chelator of zinc ion [86]. This decrease was completely blocked after culture with addition of zinc. Zinc-induced increase in bone protein synthesis was completely prevented after culture with cycloheximide or actinomycin D. Thus, bone protein synthesis has been shown to enhance with increasing age of newborn rats. Endogenous zinc in bone tissues plays a physiologic role in the enhancement of protein synthesis in bone growth [86].

Zinc has been found to stimulate the productions of IGF-I and TGF-β1 in the bone tissues of newborn rats [87]. The femoral-diaphyseal and -metaphyseal tissues were obtained at 1, 7, 14, 21, and 28 days after birth of newborn rats, and these bone tissues cultured for 24 hours in serum-free medium. The protein concentration in the culture medium was significantly increased when cultured bone tissues from newborn rats with increasing age. The medium IGF-I or TGF-β1 concentrations were gradually reduced with increasing age after birth. The presence of zinc sulfate (10^{-5} or 10^{-4} M) caused a significant increase in protein, IGF-I or TGF-β1 concentrations in culture medium. The expressions of IGF-I or TGF-β1 mRNAs were significantly increased after culture with zinc (10^{-4} M). Zinc has been shown to have stimulatory effects on IGF-I or TGF-β1 production in the femoral tissues with bone growth of newborn rats [87].

Bone growth factors are physiologically important in the stimulation of bone growth of newborn rats [88, 89]. Zinc has a physiologic role in the stimulation of bone growth in collaboration with IGF-I or TGF-β1 [90]. Culture with zinc has been shown to enhance effects of IGF-I in increasing the culture medium protein concentration, alkaline phosphatase activity or DNA content in the femoral-diaphyseal and -metaphyseal tissues obtained from newborn rats. Such an effect of zinc was not seen in case of TGF-β1. Zinc may partly regulate protein tyrosine kinase and protein tyrosine phosphatase that are related to signaling mechanism of IGF-I in the cells [68].

Zinc has been shown to stimulate *in vitro* DNA synthesis activity in the femoral-diaphyseal and -metaphyseal tissues obtained from newborn rats [91]. An increase in bone DNA synthesis activity was associated with bone growth of newborn rats with aging (1- 21 days). Bone DNA synthesis activity has been shown to reduce after culture with zinc chelator in the reaction mixture of assay system for DNA synthesis [91], indicating that bone endogenous zinc plays a role in the enhancement of bone DNA synthesis associated with bone growth of newborn rats. Also, zinc has a stimulatory effect on DNA synthesis in the femoral tissues obtained from newborn rats [91]. DNA polymerase, which is related to DNA synthesis, is a zinc enzyme. Zinc may partly stimulate DNA synthesis due to activating DNA polymerase in osteoblastic cells of bone tissues.

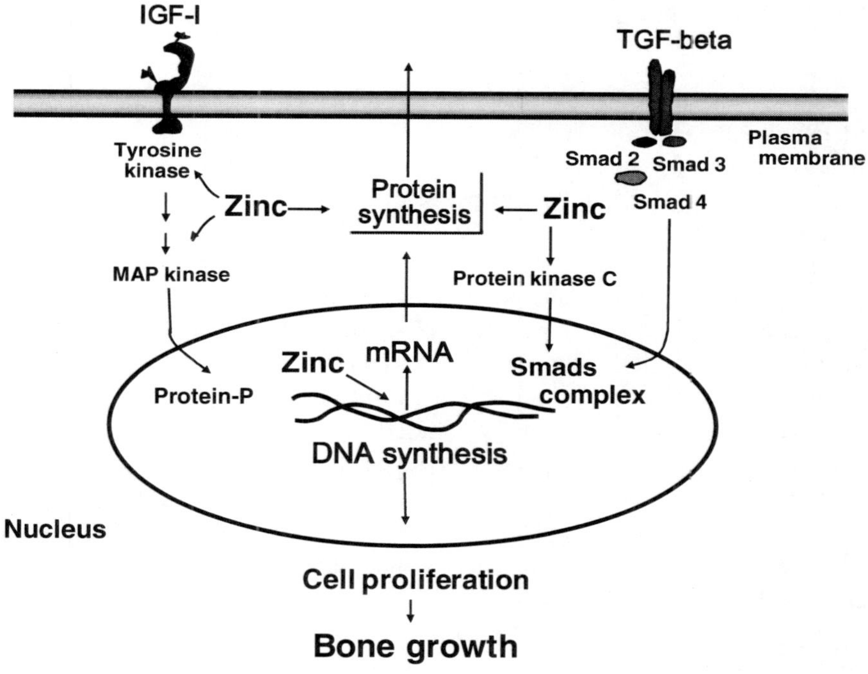

Figure 5. Cellular and molecular mechanisms by which zinc stimulates bone growth. Zinc enhances the osteogenic effects of TGF- β 1 and IGF-I in osteoblastic cells due to stimulating their signaling pathways. Zinc directly activates protein synthesis and stimulates gene expression and DNA synthesis. As the results, zinc stimulates bone growth.

Bone DNA synthesis activity is significantly increased after culture with IGF-I or TGF-β1 [91]. The effect of IGF-I in increasing bone DNA synthesis activity is found to significantly be enhanced in the presence of zinc. This effect was not seen in case of TGF-β1. The effect of zinc, IGF-I, or zinc plus IGF-I in increasing bone DNA synthesis activity was completely prevented after culture with an inhibitor of mitosis-activated protein (MAPK) kinase. Zinc has a stimulatory effect on bone DNA synthesis in newborn rats. Zinc has been demonstrated to increase the proliferation of osteoblastic MC3T3-E1 cells *in vitro* [64].

Presumably, zinc activates MAPK kinase and has a stimulatory effect on the proliferation of osteoblastic cells in the bone tissues of newborn rats [90]. Zinc deficiency has been reported to induce a decrease in serum IGF-I level and a retardation of skeletal growth in young rats [32]. Zinc may play an important role in the stimulation of bone growth in collaboration with IGF-I in newborn rats.

As mentioned above, the cellular and molecular mechanisms by which zinc stimulates bone growth in newborn rats has been shown in Figure 5.

Zinc Stimulates Fracture Healing

Fracture repair can be considered as a biologically optimal process resulting in the restoration of injured skeletal tissue to a state of normal structure and function [92]. The mechanism by which bone fracture heals is complex. Fracture healing can be envisioned as involving five distinguishable processes, including the immediate response to injury, intramembranous bone formation, chondrogenesis, endochondral bone formation leading to the reestablishment of load bearing function, and bone remodeling [92, 93]. It has been recognized that these processes may occur simultaneously during fracture repair. During fracture healing, a number of growth factors, cytokines, and their cognate receptors are present at elevated levels in and around the fracture site [94].

Zinc has been shown to stimulate fracture healing. The role of zinc in fracture healing has been determined using the diaphyseal tissues obtained at 7 or 14 days after the fracture of femoral diaphysis of rats [95-98]. The protein content in the femoral-diaphyseal tissues was markedly increased in fracture healing, and many protein molecules were produced in the bone tissues with healing [96]. When the diaphyseal tissues with fracture healing were cultured, significant increases in bone alkaline phosphatase activity and DNA content were caused. These increases were significantly enhaced after culture with zinc compound [96]. Such increases were completely prevented after culture with an inhibitor of protein synthesis.

Culture with diaphyseal tissues of fracture healing caused a significant increase in IGF-I or TGF-β1 in culture medium [97]. The production of IGF-I or TGF-β1 from bone tissues with fracture healing was significantly enhanced after culture with zinc compound. The effect of IGF-I or TGF-β1 in increasing protein content in the bone tissues with fracture healing was enhanced after culture with zinc compound [97].

When the femoral-diaphyseal tissues obtained from rats with fracture healing were cultured for 24 hours in a serum-free medium, many proteins in the bone tissues were released into the culture medium [98]. Especially, a protein molecule of approximately 66 kDa was markedly increased with fracture healing. The increase in 66 kDa molecule was enhanced after culture with zinc compound [98]. The effect of zinc in increasing the 66 kDa molecule was based on a newly synthesized protein. The production of bone osteocalcin, which is significantly increased during fracture healing, has been shown to enhance after culture with zinc compound [99].

The results of N-terminal sequencing of 66 kDa protein showed that the N-terminus is identical to that of rat albumin [99]. The expression of albumin was seen in the diaphyseal (cortical bone) and metaphyseal (trabecular bone) tissues of rat femur. The production of albumin in the bone tissues with fracture healing has been shown to increase after culture with PTH, IGF-I, or zinc compound [99]. Albumin has been demonstrated to express in bone marrow cells and osteoblastic MC3T3-E1 cells [100]. Albumin has been shown to stimulate the proliferation of osteoblastic MC3T3-E1 cells, and it suppresses alkaline phosphatase activity that is a marker enzyme of the differentiation of the cells *in vitro* [101]. Albumin has also been shown to have a suppressive effect on Runx2 (type 1) mRNA expression and a stimulatory effect on α1 (I) collagen mRNA level in osteoblastic MC3T3-E1 cells *in vitro* [102]. Albumin may play a physiologic role in bone formation and mineralization in osteoblastic cells.

Thus, fracture healing induces a remarkable production of albumin, which has an anabolic effect on bone, in the femoral-diaphyseal tissues of rats. Zinc promotes fracture healing due to increasing many bone protein components including albumin, IGF-I and TGF-β1 which can stimulate osteoblastic bone formation.

Bone fracture often occurs in osteoporosis. Chemical factors that can stimulate the healing of bone fracture have not been fully developed. The daily oral administration of zinc acexamate (100 mg Zn/kg) for 28 days caused a significant increase in calcium content, alkaline and acid phosphatase activities, protein and DNA contents in the femoral-diaphyseal tissues of rats with fracture healing [103]. Supplemental intake of zinc compound has a usefullness in promotion of fracture healing of the femoral-diaphyseal tissues in rats.

Restorative Effect of Zinc Compound on Bone Loss

β-Alanyl-L-histidinato zinc (II) (AHZ), in which zinc is chelated to β-alanyl-L-histidine, is a new zinc compound. Its molecular weight is 289.61. Oral administration of AHZ has been found to stimulate bone growth in weanling rats, and the compound has a potent effect as compared that of zinc sulfate [104]. AHZ has been demonstrated to stimulate bone formation in tissue culture [105] and proliferation and differentiation of osteoblastic cells *in vitro* [64, 65], and such effect of AHZ was potent as compared with that of zinc sulfate.

AHZ is easily absorbed from the intestine. Zinc in AHZ may largely accumulation in bone cells without difficulty because the metal binds to the hydroxyapatite of bone tissue [106]. AHZ can easily enter bone cells (osteoblasts and osteoclasts) in comparison with that of zinc sulfate [107]. This explains that AHZ has potent effects as compared to the effects of zinc sulfate on bone.

AHZ has a potent stimulatory effect on protein synthesis in osteoblastic cells [108]. Aminoacyl-tRNA synthetase is an enzyme that synthesizes aminoacyl-tRNA, and the enzyme in osteoblastic cells was directly activated by AHZ (10^{-7} to 10^{-5} M). The effect of AHZ in increasing aminoacyl-tRNA synthetase activity was greater than that of zinc sulfate [109]. AHZ may be able to bind easily to aminoacyl-tRNA synthetase. β-Alanyl-L-histidine did not have an effect. Zinc ion is required in the revelation of AHZ action, since effect of AHZ is completely abolished in the presence of dipicolinate, a chelator of zinc ion.

The effect of zinc sulfate, AHZ, di(N-acetyl-β-alanyl-L-histidinato) zinc, and di(histidino) zinc on bone metabolism has also been examined *in vivo* and *in vitro* [108, 109]. The chemical form of zinc-chelating β-alanyl-L-histidine has been demonstrated to have potent-anabolic effects on bone formation and calcification in some dipeptides used as ligand.

AHZ has been shown to have preventive effects on bone loss with various pathophysiologic conditions. Zinc content in the cellular components, but not the matrix, has been demonstrated to be lower in the femoral diaphysis of aged rats (30 weeks old) than in that of weanling rats (3 weeks old) [110, 111]. Bone protein synthesis most likely deteriorates with increasing age. Such deterioration has been found to restore after the oral administration of zinc (5 to 20 mg Zn/kg) for 3 days. The depletion of zinc in bone cells may cause deterioration of bone formation in aged rats. The decrease in bone zinc with aging may play a role in development of bone loss with increasing age. The supplementation of zinc may be important in the prevention of bone loss with aging. AHZ (10 - 75 mg/kg body weight/day) was orally administered to aged rats (30 weeks old). The administration of AHZ caused a significant increase in zinc, calcium and DNA contents in the femoral diaphysis [112]. The anabolic effects of AHZ have also been shown in the tissue culture using bone obtained from aged rats *in vitro* [113].

It has been known that skeletal unloading caused by immobilization, spaceflight, bedrest, or hindlimb suspension results in osteopenia. Zinc content has been shown to be decreased in the femoral-metaphyseal tissues of rats with skeletal unloading [114, 115]. Skeletal unloading induces an inhibition of bone formation and an increae in bone resorption, thereby decreasing in bone mass [116]. Skeletal unloading was designed using the model of hindlimb suspension in rats, which we developed. Animals were fed for 4 days with the unloading. Unloading induced a significant decresae in metaphyseal zinc content. Zinc accumulation into the metaphyseal tissues after a single oral administation of zinc sulfate (200 mg Zn/kg) was depressed after unloading [114]. The serum zinc concentration in skeletal-unloaded rats was higher than that in normal rats. The impaired movement of zinc from serum into bone tissues may be caused with unloading [114]. Skeletal unloading caused a significant decrease in bone components [114, 115]. Skeletal unloading-induced decrease in zinc content, alkaline phosphatase activity and DNA content in the femoral diaphysis of rats was restored after oral administration of AHZ (25-100 mg/kg/day) [117]. Such an effect has been shown to involve in newly synthesized proteins. The supplementation of zinc compound may have a role in the prevention of bone loss with skeletal unloading.

Aluminium has been shown to localize in the bone from patients with renal failure, and this induces bone disorders [118]. The dose of 2.7 and 5.4 mg Al/kg caused a significant increase in serum calcium concentration and bone acid phosphatase activity, while bone alkaline phosphatase activity and calcium content were not significantly altered [119]. Bone DNA content was significantly decreased with the dose of 5.4 mg Al/kg. Such decrease of bone components was completely blocked after the simultaneous administration of AHZ (10 and 25 mg/kg). AHZ can prevent the revelation of the toxic effect of aluminium on bone metabolism in rats [119].

Feeding with low-calcium and vitamin D-deficient diets induces a decrease in serum calcium concentration and a corresponding fall in bone calcium content. When rats were fed on low-calcium (0.10%) and vitamin D-deficient diets for 14 days, the decrease in serum calcium and bone calcium was observed [120]. Oral administration of AHZ (10-100 mg/kg/day) to rats fed low-calcium and vitamin D-deficient diets for 14 days resulted in an increase of bone components [120]. The serum calcium and inorganic phosphorus concentrations were not significantly altered after AHZ administration. AHZ may directly stimulate bone formation independently of alteration in serum mineral homeostasis.

The inhibition of bone formation occurs during acute inflammation in the rat, and changes in osteoblast function are part of the acute phase response following local inflammation. Bone loss is seen in rats with adjuvant arthritis; local subcutaneous injection of 1% *Mycobacterium butyricum* suspension is used to induce systemic inflammatory response in rats. The decreases in calcium content and alkaline phosphatase activity were seen in the femoral diaphysis of rats with adjuvant arthritis [121]. Oral administration of AHZ (30 and 100 mg/kg) produced a significant increase in alkaline phosphatase activity, DNA, calcium and zinc contents in the femoral tissues of rats with adjuvant arthritis. AHZ did not have a direct inhibitory effect on inflammation. AHZ (300 mg/day) treatment has been shown to improve periarticular osteoporosis, probably through an increase of bone formation, in postmenopausal women with rheumatoid arthritis [122].

Glucocorticoid therapy induces development of secondary hyperparathyroidism and the inhibition of osteoblastic function [123]. The steroid treatment caused a significant increase in serum PTH level, while serum calcium, inorganic phosphorus and zinc concentrations were not significantly altered [124]. The femoral-diaphyseal alkaline phosphatase activity, DNA and calcium contents were significantly decreased after the administration of steroid, although bone zinc content was not significantly changed. When AHZ (30 or 100 mg/kg) was orally administered for 30 days to rats administered with the steroid, the administration completely prevented increase in serum PTH levels and decrease in the bone components caused by the steroid treatment. Bone zinc content was significantly increased after the administration of AHZ. AHZ may have a therapeutic effect in steroid-induced osteoporosis.

Ovariectomy causes a lack of estrogen. Estrogen deficiency induces osteoporosis in humans and in rats [125, 126]. Ovariectomy caused a significant decrease in alkaline phosphatase activity, DNA and calcium contents in the femoral diaphysis of rats [127-129]. These decreases were completely prevented after oral administration of AHZ (10-100 mg/kg/day) for 6 weeks [127]. AHZ restored bone loss in ovariectomized rats. Moreover, rats were fed for 3 weeks after ovariectomy, and then the animals were orally administered AHZ (10-100 mg/kg/day) for 3 months [103, 104]. A remarkable decrease in estrogen concentration in rat serum was seen 3 months after ovariectomy. Prolonged oral administration of AHZ did not influence serum estrogen level after ovariectomy. The administration of AHZ completely prevented the reduction of bone mass [128]. The administration of AHZ for 3 months could completely prevent reduction in mineral content in the trabecular and cortical bone tissues of ovariectomized rats [129]. AHZ has been shown to have a preventive effect on ovariectomy-induced bone loss.

Zinc acexamate [zinc 6-(acetylamino)hexanoate] has been shown to have a potent effect on bone formation as compared with that of zinc sulafate and AHZ *in vitro* [130]. Zinc acexamate may be a good tool in therapy of osteoporosis. Bone loss has been shown to induce with diabetes [131, 132]. Streptozotocin (STZ)-diabetic rats induce an impairment of insulin secretion. A single subcutaneous administration of STZ (60 mg/kg body weight) to rats caused a significant decrease in body weight and serum zinc concentration, a remarkable increase in serum glucose and triglyceride levels, and a significant decrease in alkaline phosphatase activity, calcium and DNA contents in the femoral-diaphyseal and -metaphyseal tissues of STZ-diabetic rats [133, 134]. Zinc acexamate (25 mg Zn/kg) was orally administered once daily for 14 or 21 days to rats received a single subcutaneous administration of STZ. Zinc acexamate had potent-preventive effects on the changes in body weight, serum findings and bone loss in STZ-administered rats, indicating that the compound has restorative effects in insulin-dependent (Type I) diabetic conditions [132, 134]. Zinc acexamate had a potent-preventive effect on diabetic conditions as compared with zinc sulfate. Zinc acexamate may have preventive and therapeutic effects on diabetes-induced bone loss in rats.

In addition, citrated zinc bisglycinate has been developed as a zinc supplement. This compound has been shown to increase bioavailability in intestinal absorption of zinc, and it is used as a zinc supplementation.

Involvment of Zinc in Osteoporosis

Osteoporotic patients have been shown to have lower levels of skeletal zinc than healthy individuals [46]. The reduction of levels of biological markers of nutrition in postmenopausal osteoporosis may be related to zinc deficiency. In postmenopausal women, urinary zinc has been used as a marker of bone resorption. The plasma and urinary zinc concentrations in 30 women with postmenopausal osteoporosis have been compared in 30 healthy postmenopausal women who served as controls [135]. The plasma zinc levels did not differ between groups, but urinary zinc excretion has been found to be significantly higher in the women with postmenopausal osteoporosis [135]. The elevation of urinary zinc elimination in osteoporosis may be dependent on bone resorption [135], because zinc is located richely in bone tissues. The measurement of urinary zinc may be a useful biochemical method of observing the positive clinical effect following alendronate or calcitonin therapy in postmenopausal women [136].

The relationship between indices of zinc nutritive status and biochemical markers of bone turnover in older adult European subjects has been shown [137]. A total of 387 healthy adults, aged 55-87 years are used in this study. There was seen some, albeit inconsistent, evidence of a relationship between zinc nutritive status and bone turnover in the older adult participants of the ZENITH study [137].

The supplements of trace minerals with or without calcium in postmenopausal women have been shown to have beneficial effects on bone density [138]. Low zinc intakes and reduced blood zinc concentrations have been reported to be associated with osteoporosis in women [138]. To examine the independent association between dietary zinc and plasma zinc and the association of each with bone mineral density and 4 years-bone loss in community-dwelling older men, of the original Rancho Bernardo Study subjects, 396 men (age: 45-92 years) were used. The mean dietary zinc intake was 11.2 mg. Dietary zinc intake and plasma zinc each have a positive association with BMD in men [138].

Protein undernutrition is frequent in the elderly. It contributes to the development of osteoporosis, possibly via lower IGF-I. Dietary zinc can influence IGF-I production. In the elder, zinc supplementation accelerated the serum IGF-I response to essential amino acids-whey protein supplements by 1 week and decreased a biochemical marker of bone resorption [139].

The changes in circulating biochemical markers of bone metabolism in aged individuals with food intake supplemented with zinc have been examined [140]. Sixty-three volunteers (31 men and 32 women) were divided into four groups of 15 or 16 male volunteers and 16 or 16 female volunteers, and each group was sequentially food containing 0.8 mg or 3.6 mg zinc once a day for 4 or 8 weeks as follows. The dietary intake of zinc for 8 weeks in men or women caused a significant increase in serum bone-specific alkaline phosphatase activity and γ-carboxylated osteocalcin concentration and a significant decrease in serum bone TRACP activity and N-telopeptide of type I collagen, as compared with the control group without dietary zinc [140]. This study suggests that supplementation with zinc has stimulatory effects on bone formation and suppressive effects on bone resorption in aged individuals. Thus, the intake of dietary zinc may have benefit effects in the prevention and treatment of osteoporosis.

Conclusion

Nutritional zinc is abundant in bone and may act as a local regulator of bone cells. Zinc plays a physiologic role in the regulation of bone homeostasis. Zinc stimulates osteoblastic bone formation and mineralization and inhibits osteoclastic bone resorption, thereby increasing bone mass [141-144]. Various zinc-related regulatory proteins have been identified in bone cells. Zinc tranporter, zinc finger-containing transcription factor, called Osterix (Osx), Cas-interacting zinc finger protein (CIZ), a novel type inhibitor of bone morphogenetic protein (BMP)/Smad signaling, Schnurri-3 (Shn3), a mammalian homolog of the Drosophila zinc finger adapter protein Shn, has been found in osteoblastic cells and osteoclastic cells. Moreover, intracellular zinc stimulates the synthesis of many proteins at translational process due to activating aminoacyl-tRNA synthetase and to stimulate gene expressions in osteoblastic cells. Zinc also increases DNA synthesis in the cells. Thus, zinc has been shown to have an important role in the regulation of osteoblasts and osteoclasts. Zinc deficiency may attenuate function of these bone cells.

The decrease in bone zinc with pathophysiologic state has been shown to lead bone loss. The supplemental intake of zinc prevents and treats bone loss. Zinc yeast has been shown to have a high bioavailability in rats and its dietary intake has anabolic effects on bone components *in vivo* [145], indicating its usefulness as a functional food ingredient. Also, zinc-binding aminoacid compounds are usefulness. β-Alanyl-L-histidinato zinc (AHZ) or zinc acexamate has been shown to have a potent anabolic effect in comparison with zinc sulfate. In addition, citrated zinc bisglycinate has been developed as a zinc supplement. These compounds may be a clinical usefulness in therapy of osteoporosis. Zinc supplementation may play an important role in the prevention and treatment of osteoporosis.

Chapter 3

Dietary Soybean Genistein and Osteoporosis Treatment

Osteoporosis with its accompanying decrease in bone mass is widely recognized as a major public health problem. Malnutrition or undernutrition is often observed in the elderly, and it appears to be more intense in patients with hip fracture than in the general aging population. The deficiency in both micronutrients and macronutrients appears to be strongly implicated in the pathogenesis and the consequences of hip fracture in the osteoporotic elderly. Isoflavones (including daidzin, daidzein, genistein, and genistein) are contained in soybeans with relatively high concentrations. Daidzin or genistin is hydrolyzed to daidzein or genistein by β-glucosidase in the gastrointestinal system, respectively (Figure 6). Genistein has been found to have a strong inhibitory effect on protein tyrosine kinase and it can cause cell cycle arrest and apotosis in leukemic cells [146]. This cellular mechanism of genistein may be important in prevention of cancers.

The author *et al.* found that genistein or daidzein has been demonstrated to have a direct anabolic effect on bone metabolism *in vitro* [147], suggesting a role in the prevention of osteoporosis. This was the first time finding. Genistein, which is contained in soybeans, has been shown to have a stimulatory effect on osteoblastic bone formation and a suppressive effect on osteoclastic bone resorption, thereby increasing bone mass. This factor has regulatory effects on protein synthesis and gene expression, which are related to bone formation in osteoblastic cells and bone resorption in osteoclastic cells. Oral administration of genistein has been shown to prevent on bone loss in ovariectomized rats, an animal model for osteoporosis, indicating a role in the prevention of osteoporosis. Moreover, the intake of dietary soybean genistein has been shown to have a restorative effect on osteoporosis in human subjects, suggesting a role in the treatment of bone loss. Genistein is as a biomedical food factor, which is useful in the prevention and treatment of osteoporosis.

This chapter introduces the role of soybean genistein in the regulation of bone homeostasis and in the prevention and treatment of osteoporosis in animal models and human subjects.

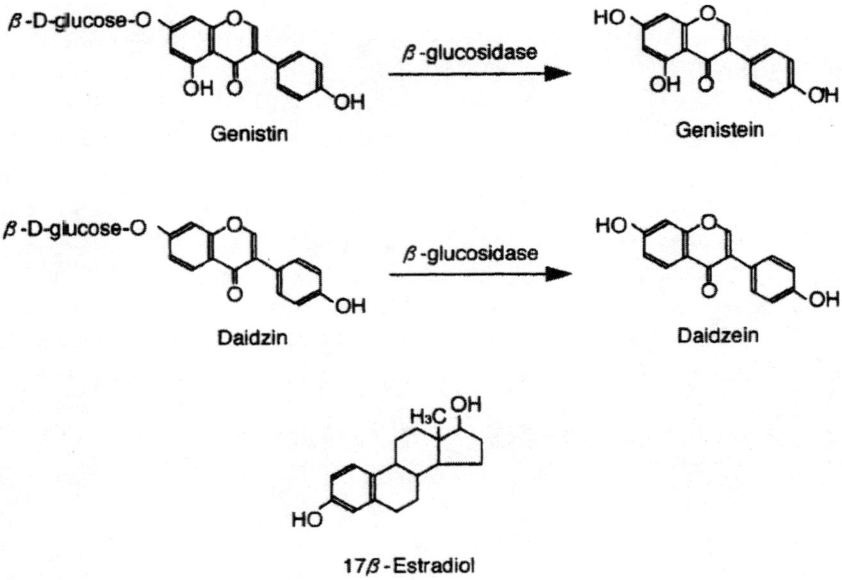

Figure 6. Chemical structure of isoflavones. Genistin and daidzin are hydrolyzed to daidzein and genistein by β-glucosidase in the gastrointestinal system, respectively.

Genistein Stimulates Osteoblastic Bone Formation

Genistein Has Anabolic Effects in Bone Tissues

The anabolic effects of genistein on bone metabolism have initiately been demonstrated in tissue culture using the femoral metaphyseal (trabecular bone) tissues obtained from elderly female rats *in vitro* [147, 148]. Bone tissues were cultured for 24 hours in a Dulbecco's modified Eagle's medium (high glucose, 4.5%) with bovine serum albumin (serum free) containing either vehicle or genistein. The presence of genistein (10^{-6} or 10^{-5} M) caused a significant increase in bone components (calcium content, alkaline phosphatase activity and DNA content) in rat femoral metaphyseal tissues [147, 148]. The effect of genistein in increasing bone components is equal to the stimulatory effects of 17β-estradiol, which is important as anabolic hormone in bone metabolism. Anti-estrogen agent tamoxifen inhibited genistein-induced increase in bone components, although tamoxifen itself had no effect on bone components [147]. Anabolic effects of genistein on bone metabolism may be partly mediated through estrogen-like action. Presumably, genistein binds to the receptor of estrogen in osteoblastic cells in which the receptor is localized [149].

The effects of genistein or genistin on bone components have been compared in *in vitro* culture system [147]. Culture with genistein (10^{-8} - 10^{-5} M) or genistin (10^{-7} - 10^{-5} M) increased alkaline phosphatase activity and DNA and calcium contents in the femoral-metaphyseal tissues obtained from elderly female rats [147]. The effect of genistein was greater than that of genistin. The effects of genistein or genistin in increasing bone components were blocked in the presence of cycloheximide, an inhibitor of protein synthesis in the translational process, suggesting that anabolic effects of the isoflavones are partly resulted from newly synthesized protein components.

The anabolic effects of daizein on the femoral-diaphyseal (cortical bone) tissues obtained from elderly female rats *in vitro* have also been shown [150]. The presence of daidzein (10^{-6} or 10^{-5} M) in culture medium caused a significant increase in bone components. The effect of daizein was equal to that of genistein (10^{-6} or 10^{-5} M). Combination of daidzein and genistein did not have an additive effect [150]. In addition, the stimulatory effects of daidzein on bone components were completely suppressed in presence of cycloheximide [150], suggesting that such effect is resulted from protein synthsis.

The effects of phosphogenistein and phosphodaidzein, which are phosphorylated for the hydroxyl group at the 7-position of genistein and daidzein, on bone components has been compared to the effect of genistein or daizen [151]. Phosphogenistein or phosphodaidzein increased bone components in tissue culture *in vitro*. Phosphoisoflavones with a lower concentration of 10^{-6} M, at which genistein and daidzein have anabolic effects on bone components, did not have an effect [151].

The effects of various polyphenols found in food and plants on bone metabolism have also been compared [152]. Glycitein, resveratol, quercetin, catechin, and (-)-epigallocatechin gallate did not have an anabolic effect on bone calcification *in vitro* [152]. Polyphenols did not have a direct stimulatory effect on bone calcification *in vitro*. Among various polyphenol, genistein has unique anabolic effects on bone.

As mentioned above, genistein is a 4', 5, 7-trihydroxyisoflavone, and daidzein is a 4', 7-dihydroxyisoflavone. Glycitein is a 4', 7-dihydroxy-6-methoxyflavone, while quercetin is a 3, 3', 4', 5, 7-pontahydeoxyflavone; neither has any effects of genistein and daidzein on bone calcification is weakened by the phosphorylation of the hydroxy-group at their-7-position [152]. The hydroxy-groups at the 5- and 7-positions of the isoflavone genistein may be necessary for its anabolic effect on bone formation, suggesting a chemical structure-activity relationship. Presumably, the chemical form of dihydroxyisoflavone is important to have anabolic effects on bone. Genistein and daidzein may have bone effects that are partly mediated through the same mechanism.

Genistein Stimulates Osteoblastogenesis

Osteoblasts play an essential role in the stimulation of bone formation and calcification. The anabolic effects of isoflavones on osteoblastic cells *in vitro* have been demonstrated [153-155]. Osteoblastic MC3T3-E1 cells were cultured for 48 hours in a serum-free modified Eagle's medium containing genistein or daidzein. The presence of genistein (10^{-6} or 10^{-5} M) or daidzein (10^{-6} or 10^{-5} M) caused a significant increase in protein content, alkaline phosphatase activity and DNA content in the cells [153]. The ability of genistein or daidzein to increase biochemical components in the cells was not seen in the presence of an inhibitor of protein synthesis [153], suggesting that the effects of isoflavones result from newly synthesized protein components. The anabolic effects of genistein in osteoblastic cells are not distinguishable from those of daidzein [153, 154].

The effects of 17β-estradiol in increasing protein content and alkaline phosphatase activity in osteoblastic cells were not enhanced in the presence of genistein [153]. Cellular protein content was additively increased with 17β-estradiol and daidzein, but their effects on alkaline phosphatase activity were not additively. The receptors of estrogen are found in osteoblastic cells. Genistein has been shown to bind to estrogen receptor β in osteoblastic cells [149], and daidzein cannot bind to the receptor [149]. It has been speculated that genistein may bind to estrogen receptor β in osteoblastic cells, although the nuclear localization of genistein in these cells has poorly understood.

DNA content in osteoblastic cells was increased in the presence of genistein or daizein, suggesting that isoflavones stimulate cell proliferation [153, 154]. Isoflavones increase alkaline phosphatase activity, which is a marker enzyme in differentiation of osteoblastic cells. Genistein and daidzein may have stimulatory effects on the proliferation and differentiation of osteoblastic MC3T3-E1 cells.

The cellular mechanism by which isoflavones stimulate osteoblastic bone formation has been studied in relation to protein synthesis [155]. The presence of genistein or daidzein stimulated protein synthesis in osteoblastic MC3T3-E1 cells *in vitro* [155]. The addition of genistein or daidzein into the reaction mixture has been shown to cause a significant increase in *in vitro* protein synthesis using the cell homogenate obtained from osteoblastic cells cultured without isoflavone [155]. Such an increase was suppressed in the presence of an inhibitor of protein synthesis, indicating that genistein or daidzein can directly stimulate protein synthesis *in vitro*. Moreover, genistein or daidzein has been shown to increase [^{3}H]-leucyl-tRNA synthetase activity in the cytosol fraction of osteoblastic cell homogenate [155]. Genistein had a greater effect than daidzein [155]. Thus, the isoflavone can directly activate leucyl-tRNA synthetase, a rate-limiting enzyme in the translational process of protein synthesis.

The possibility, that genistein or daidzein acts on the translational process in osteoblastic MC3T3-E1 cells, cannot exclude, since the stimulatory effects of the isoflavones on protein synthesis in osteoblastic cells are suppressed by actinomycin D, an inhibitor of transcription activity [155]. Genistein has been shown to bind to estrogen receptors in osteoblastic cells [149], although daidzein cannot bind to estrogen receptors [149]. Moreover, it is possible that genistein or daidzein can bind to other transcription factors, which differ from estrogen receptors, in osteoblastic MC3T3-E1 cells.

The estrogenic compounds of 17β-estradiol and genistein mediate very different actions on osteoblastic cells [156]. While 17β-estradiol may stimulate bone anabolism, in part, by antagonizing TNFα-induced NF-κB activation, genistein did not only fail to prevent the cytokin-induced NF-κB activation, but directly promotes NF-κB activation in MC3T3 cells [156]. These observations suggest an important mechanistic difference in the mechanisms by which 17β-estradiol and genistein promote osteoblast differentiation [156]. Whether genistein has an effect on various protein kinases and protein phosphatases which are related to osteoblastic cell proliferation and nuclear transcription activity remains to be elucidated.

Molecular Mechanism by Which Genistein Stimulates Osteoblastogenesis

The cellular and molecular mechanisms by which genistein enhances osteoblastogenesis have been investigated [157, 158]. Culture with genistein (10^{-5} M) has been found to have stimulatory effects on the mineralization in osteoblastic cells *in vitro* [157]. Alkaline phosphatase is an enzyme marker of osteoblasts and the enzyme participates in bone mineralization [158]. α1 (I) collagen is a matrix protein that is related to bone formation and mineralization in osteoblast lineage cells [159]. Osteocalcin, which is synthesized in osteoblasts, is a bone matrix protein containing γ_2-carboxyglutamin acid and is involved in mineralization [159]. The expression of alkaline phosphatase, α1 (I) collagen, and osteocalcin mRNAs in osteoblastic cells was markedly enhanced after culture with genistein (10^{-6} or 10^{-5} M) as compared to the effect of each factor [157].

The effect of genistein (10^{-5} M) on the gene expressions in osteoblastic cells was completely depressed in the presence of cycloheximide, an inhibitor of protein synthesis, and 5, 6-dichlorobenzimidazone-1-β-D-ribofuranoside (DRB), an inhibitor of transcriptional activity [157]. These findings suggest that genistein stimulates transcriptional process in osteoblastic cells. Genistein may have a stimulatory effect on protein synthesis at the transcriptional process. Genistein (10^{-6} or 10^{-5} M) was found to increase protein content in osteoblastic MC3T3-E1 cells *in vitro* [157]. Such effect may involve in the activation of aminoacyl-tRNA synthase, a rate-limiting enzyme in protein synthesis. Genistein may stimulate both transcriptional and translational activities in osteoblastic cells. Genistein may have an effect on the binding of transcriptional factor(s), which is synthesized through translational process, to the nuclear DNA in osteoblastic cells.

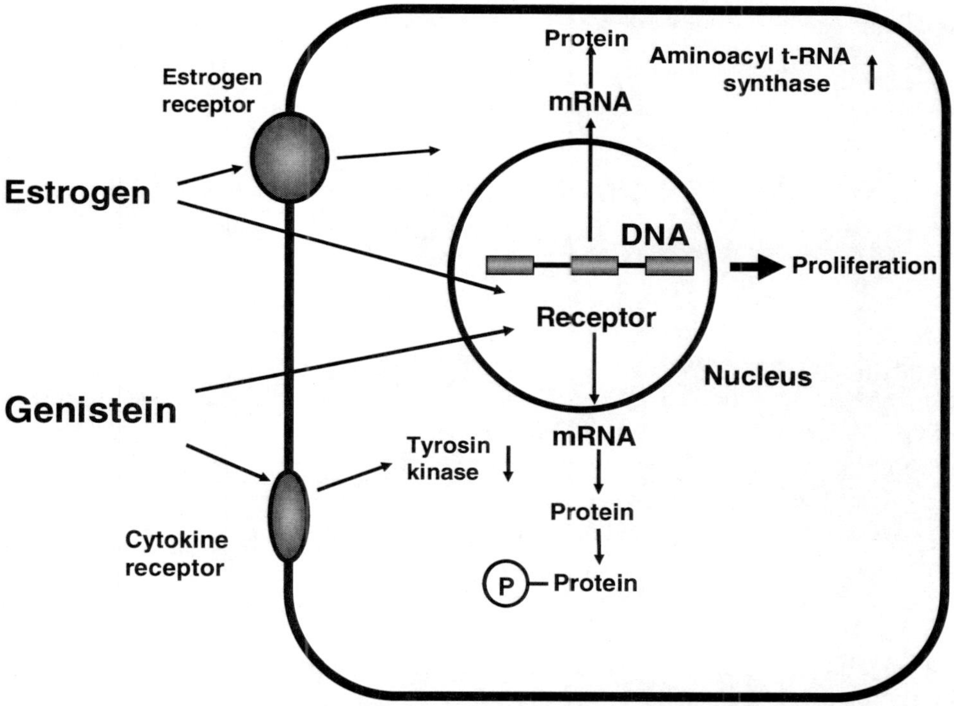

Figure 7. Molecular and cellular mechanisms by which genistein stimulates osteoblastic bone formation. Genistein directly activates aminiacyl-tRNA synthase, a rate-limiting enzyme in translational process, in osteoblastic cells. Genistein can increase protein synthesis and also may be able to enhance transcriptional activity by its binding to estrogen receptors and/or its direct effect on gene in the cells.

Genistein (10^{-6} M) has been shown to result in an increase in cell proliferation and stimulate osteoblastic maturation as assessed by culture duration-dependent increments in alkaline phosphatase activity, calcium deposition into extracellular matrix and Runx2/Cbfa1 gene expression in primary mouse bone marrow-derived mesenchymal stem cells (BMSCs) cultures [160]. Genistein also resulted in an increase in nitric oxide (NO) synthase activity, NO formation, and cyclic guanosine 3', 5'-monophosphate production in BMSCs cultures [160]. These effects of genistein were mimicked by 17β-estradiol [160].

Whether genistein and daidzein regulate target gene transcription through cyclic adenosine 3', 5'-monophosphate (cAMP) regulatory element (CRE) in human osteoblastic cell line MG-63 cells has been shown [161]. It has been found that 17β-estradiol, genistein and daidzein suppressed the transcriptional activity of CRE-luciferase reporter gene in MG-63 cells [161]. 17β-Estradiol and genistein but not daidzein inhibited the cAMP analogue 8-Br cAMP-induced transcription of CRE reporter gene [161]. Both genistein and 17β-estradiol inhibited basal and cAMP-induced mRNA levels of endogenous estrogen responsive genes containing CRE/CRE-like elements in their promoter regions, including interleukin (IL) 8 and serum- and glucocorticoid-inducible kinase 1 [161]. These findings indicate that genistein and daidzein may modulate bone remodeling through ERs by regulating target gene expression through the CRE motifs.

The molecular and cellular mechanisms by which genistein stimulates osteoblastic bone formation are summarized in Figure 7.

Genistein Suppresses Osteoclastic bone Resorption

Genistein Suppresses Bone Resorption in Bone Tissues

Parathyroid hormone (PTH), prostaglandin E_2 (PGE_2) and lipopolysaccharide (LPS) have stimulatory effects on bone resorption in culture system *in vitro* [162 - 164]. Culture with PTH, PGE_2 or LPS clearly stimulated bone resorption in the femoral-metaphyseal tissues cultured for 48 hours when bone resorption was estimated with a decrease in bone calcium content [165]. The effects of bone-resorbing factors were completely suppressed in the presence of genistein, indicating an inhibition of bone resorption [165].

PTH and PGE_2 caused remarkable increases in glucose consumption and lactic acid production by bone tissues [165]. The production of lactic acid by bone tissues may be partly related to augmentation of glucose consumption. Presumably, PTH- and PGE_2-stimulated lactic acid productions in the bone tissues lead to a decrease in bone calcium content. Genistein completely depressed PTH- or PGE_2-induced increase in both glucose consumption and lactic acid production in bone tissues [165]. The suppressive effects of genistein on bone resorption may be partly related to prevention of lactic acid production by bone tissues.

Thus, genistein has stimulatory effects on both bone formation and mineralization in tissue culture *in vitro* and has also been found to have suppressive effects on bone resorption in tissue culture. Genistein may have an important role in preservation of bone mass.

Genistein Suppresses Osteoclastogenesis in Bone Marrow Cells

Osteoclasts, bone-resorbing cells, are formed from bone marrow stem cells [8, 9]. Osteoclast-like cell formation is estimated using staining for tartrate-resistant acid phosphatase (TRACP), a marker enzyme of osteoclasts [166]. Mouse bone marrow cells were cultured for 7 days in a medium containing a bone-resorbing agent [PTH, PGE_2, 1, 25-dihydroxyvitamin D_3 [1, $25(OH)_2D_3$], or LPS] with an effective concentration [166]. Culture with PTH, PGE_2, 1, $25(OH)_2D_3$, or LPS induced a remarkable increase in osteoclast-like multinucleated cells. These increases were depressed in the presence of genistein [167]. Suppressive effects of genistein (10^{-5} M) were equal to effects of other anti-bone-resorbing agents (calcitonin, 17β-estradiol, and zinc sulfate) on osteoclast-like cell formation in mouse marrow culture [167].

Genistein has been shown to have a potent-suppressive effect at the later stage of differentiation of bone marrow cells [167]. The suppressive effects of genistein on osteoclast-like MNC formation in mouse bone marrow culture were greater than that of daidzein. The suppressive effect of genistein on osteoclast-like MNC formation induced by PTH or PGE_2 may be partly based on the blocking of the pathway of cyclic AMP signaling, but not that by protein kinase C signaling, at the differentiation stage of bone marrow cells [167]. In addition, if genistein can inhibit tyrosine kinase [146], the action of isoflavone on osteoclastic cell formation may be partly related to its inhibitory effect on the kinase. Cellular mechanism by which genistein inhibits osteoclast-like cell formation from marrow cells may also be involved in cyclic AMP signaling.

Interleukin-6 (IL-6) has been known to stimulate osteoclastogenesis, and osteoprotegerin (OPG) depress binding of RANKL to RANK, which is receptor protein of RANKL [8, 9]. These factors are produced in osteoblastic cells [8, 9]. OPG mRNA expression has been found to increase in osteoblastic cells treated with 17β-estradiol, genistein, or daidzein [168]. The release of IL-6 in the cells was suppressed, while OPG production was enhanced by isoflavone treatments [168]. After addition of estrogen receptor-binding blocker, ICI-182780, the effects of isoflavones on OPG and IL-6 production disappeared [168]. Thus, the inhibition of IL-6 production and stimulation of OPG with dietary isoflavones may be mediated, at least in part, via a genomic pathway operating through estrogen receptors and gene expression mechanisms [168]. The stimulation of OPG mRNA expression with genistein was not affected by protein synthesis inhibitor, cycloheximide [169]. This stimulation may be involved in enhancement of OPG gene transcription [169]. Thus, genistein may partly suppress bone loss, which are mediated through enhanced the production of OPG in osteoblastic cells.

RANKL or tumor necrosis factor-α (TNF-α) has been shown to stimulate osteoclastic differentiation using RAW264.7, a murine monocytic cell line. The direct effects of estrogen on osteoclast precursor differentiation has been shown that, in addition to effecting osteoblasts, estrogen may protect bone by reducing osteoclast production [170]. The both genistein and estrogen has been found to inhibit RANKL-induced IkappaB degradation and NF-kappaB (NF-κB) nuclear localization, which is an intracellular signaling factor of RANKL, with the same relative potency as seen in proliferation and differentiation assays [171]. Genistein has been shown to depress TNF-α-induced c-fos and NFATc1 expressions in an estrogen receptor-dependent manner and also inhibit NFATc1 nuclear translocation [172].

This finding suggests that genistein suppresses TNF-α-induced osteoclastogenesis via inhibition of c-fos-dependent NFATc1 expression [172].

Genistein Suppresses Mature Osteoclasts

Genistein has been found to induce cell death (apoptosis) of osteoclasts isolated from rat femoral tissues [173, 174]. Calcitonin has been known to inhibit osteoclast activity [175]. This hormonal effect may be mediated through the two pathways of cyclic AMP and Ca^{2+} signalings. The addition of dibucaine, an antagonist of calmodulin, or staurosporine, an inhibitor of pretin kinase C, completely prevented the decrease in osteoclasts induced by calcitonin, dibutyryl cyclic AMP or calcium chloride [173]. The effect of genistein in decreasing osteoclasts was clearly suppressed by these inhibitors, suggesting that the effect of isoflavones on mature osteoclasts is partly mediated through the pathway of Ca^{2+} signaling.

A Ca^{2+} ionophore (A23187) caused a remarkable decrease in the number of osteoclasts, indicating that the entry of Ca^{2+} in the cells induces death of osteoclasts [176]. The number of osteoclasts was decreased when were cultured in the presence of genistein or calcium chloride. Ca^{2+} can activate endonuclease and induces apoptosis in the cells [177]. The effect of A23187 in decreasing osteoclasts may be based on Ca^{2+}-activated DNA fragmentation, which induces apoptosis. Genistein has been shown to induce apoptosis in immature human thymocytes by inhibiting torosisomerase II [178].

Genistein may stimulate apoptosis of osteoclasts, and its mechanism is partly related to the pathway of Ca^{2+} signaling. It is possible that genistein stimulates Ca^{2+} entry into osteoclasts, since it has been reported that the isoflavone can directly open a chloride channel in human cystic fibrosis transmembranes [173]. In addition, daidzein has also been shown to suppress the number of mature osteoclasts [173], although daidzein did not have a greater suppressive effect than genistein. The effect of daidzein was abolished in the presence of dibucaine or staurosporine, supporting a partial involvement in Ca^{2+}-signaling mechanism [173].

Culture with genistein has been found to cause an inhibition of protein kinase activity and an increase in protein tyrosine phosphatase activity in osteoclasts [174]. Genistein has a strong inhibitory effect on protein tyrosine kinases [146]. The inhibition of these kinases may induce apoptosis in a human ovarian tumor cell line and in Jurket T-leukemia cells [146]. Genistein may partly induce apoptosis of osteoclasts through a mechanism that inhibits protein tyrosine kinases in the cells. It has been shown that tyrosine kinase Src is implicated in the process of osteoclast-induced bone resorption *in vitro* and *in vivo* [179].

Culture with genistein has also been found to cause a significant increase in protein tyrosine phosphatase activity in osteoclasts [174]. This effect was also seen after addition of genistein into the enzyme reaction mixture *in vitro* [174]. Genistein can directly activate protein tyrosine phosphatase in osteoclasts. Vanadate is an inhibitor of protein tyrosine phosphatase [180]. Culture of osteoclasts in the presence of vanadate did not cause a decrease in the number of osteoclasts. The suppressive effects of genistein on osteoclasts were also seen in the presence of vanadate [174]. It has been known that protein tyrosine phosphatase (Src homology 2 domain-containing tyrosine phosphatase) is a negative regulator of osteoclastogenesis and osteoclast-resorbing activity in mutant mice [180]. Suppressive effects of genistein on mature osteoclasts may partly be mediated through the activation of protein tyrosine phosphatase in the cells.

β-Glucuronidase is a lysomal enzyme, which is involved in stimulation of bone resorption by PTH. Genistein did not have an effect on β-glucuronidase activity in osteoclasts [174]. Suppressive effects of genistein on osteoclastic bone resorption may not be implicated in the activity of lysosomal enzymes in the cells.

Thus, the suppressive effects of genistein on rat bone osteoclasts may be involved in cell apoptosis mediated through the Ca^{2+} siganaling mechanism, inhibition of protein kinase, and activation of protein tyrosine phosphatase in the cells.

Genistein Regulates Gene Expression in Osteoclasts

Genistein has been shown to regulate the gene expression of proteins that are related to osteoclast function. Culture with genistein (10^{-6} M) caused an increase in DNA fragmentation in isolated osteoclastic cells [182], indicating that genistein stimulates apoptotic cell death. In addition, genistein-induced cell death was significantly prevented in the presence of caspase-3 inhibitor [182]. However, this effect was partial. Apoptotic cell death with genistein is partly mediated through the activation of caspase-3, and also other mechanisms may participate in apoptotic cell death.

The stimulatory effects of genistein (10^{-6} M) on caspase-3 mRNA expression were completely suppressed after culture with cycloheximide, an inhibitor of protein synthesis, or DRB, an inhibitor of transcriptional activity, in osteoclastic cells with or without macrophage colony stimulating factor (M-CSF) and RANKL [50]. This finding suggests that the effect of genistein on caspase-3 mRNA expression is involved in protein synthesis and transcription activation in osteoclastic cells.

RANK activation by binding of RANKL on preosteoclasts stimulates the NF-κB signaling, propbably through association with TRAF-6 in osteoclasts [183, 184]. RANKL signaling targets include mitosis-activated protein kinases (MAPKs), NF-κB, and nuclear factor of activated T cells c1 (NFATc1) in osteoclast differentiation [183, 184]. Culture with genistein (10^{-6} M) did not cause a significant change in NF-κB mRNA expression in osteoclastic cells in the presence or absence of M-CSF and RANKL [182]. NFATc1 mRNA expression was significantly increased after culture with genistein (10^{-6} M) in osteoclastic cells cultured in the presence of M-CSF and RANKL [182]. Genistein may affect on the gene expression of NFATc1 that is a target protein of RANKL signaling in osteoclastic cells. The decrease in NFATc1 expression with the combination of genistein may be important in the revelation of suppressive effects on osteoclastogenesis and osteoclastic cell function.

The activation of TRACP or cathepsin K plays a role in promotion of osteoclastic bone resorption by stimulating the decomposition of bone matrix [182]. Genistein (10^{-6} M) did not have a significant effect on TRACP mRNA expression in osteoclastic cells [182]. Culture with genistein was found to induce a significant decrease in cathepsin K mRNA expression in osteoclastic cells cultured in the presence or absence of M-CSF and RANKL [182]. This finding demonstrates that genistein (10^{-6} M) has a suppressive effect on the activity of cathepsin K in osteoclastic cells, which are activated through RANKL signaling. Genistein has a potent-suppressive effect on bone-resorbing activity.

As described above, the suppressive effects of genistein on osteoclastic bone resorption may be involved in the inhibition of protein kinase and the activation of protein tyrosine phosphatase and the regulation of the gene expression of proteins, which are related to osteoclastic cell functions, and stimulation of cell apoptosis mediated through the Ca^{2+} siganaling mechanism. The cellular and molecular mechanisms by which genistein suppresses osteoclastic bone resorption are summarized in Figure 8.

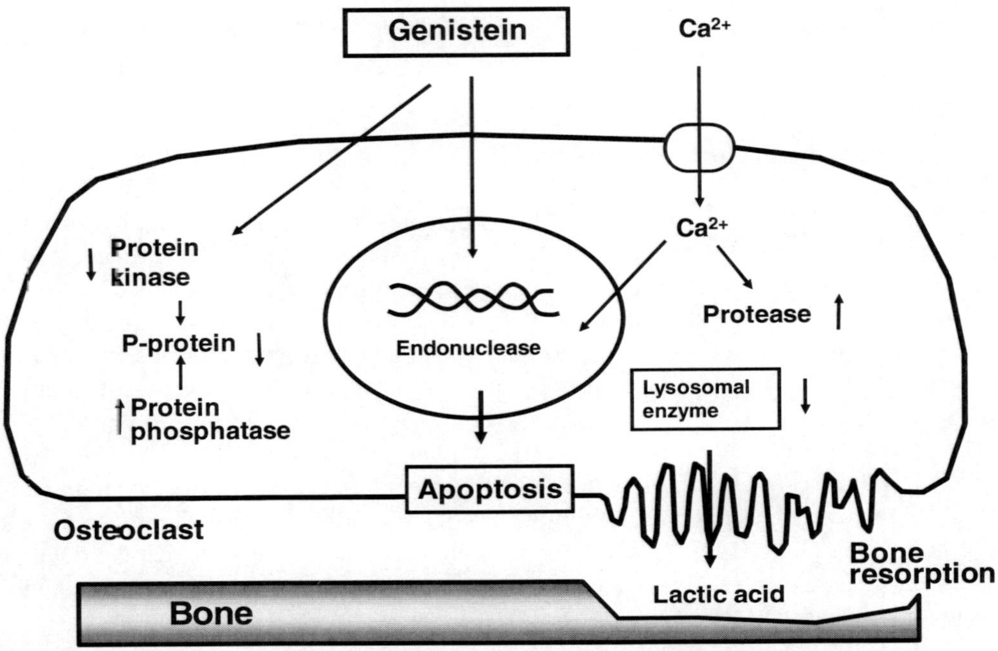

Figure 8. Cellular and molecular mechanisms by which genistein suppresses osteoclastic bone resorption. Genistein stimulates Ca^{2+} entry into osteoclasts and induces apoptosis related to Ca^{2+} signaling. Genistein inhibits protein kinase and activates protein phosphatases in osteoclasts and suppresses osteoclastic function. In addition, genistein regulates the gene expression of proteins that are related to osteoclastic functions.

Intake of Dietary Soybean Genistein Prevents Osteoporosis in Animal Model

Bone mass decreases with age. Osteoporosis with a decrease in bone mass is widely recognized as a major public health problem. This decrease may be due to increased osteoclastic bone resorption and to decreased osteoblastic bone formation. Soybean genistein has been found to stimulate osteoblastic bone formation and inhibit osteoclastic bone resorption. Whether intake of dietary soybean genistein can reveal an anabolic effect on bone *in vivo* has been demonstrated.

Nijiru, which is a by-product in the fermentation process of soybean to make fermented soybean (*natto*), contains large quantities of natural isoflavone [183]. *Nijiru* may be a functional food factor as a dietary isoflavone. Oral administration of the isoflavone-containing soybean extract (*nijiru*) to rats caused a significant increase in bone components (alkaline phosphatase activity, DNA and calcium contents) in the femoral-diaphyseal and -metaphyseal tissues *in vivo* [183], indicating the extract has an anabolic effect on bone metabolism. Also, *Nijiru* largely contains soybean saponin [184]. In addition, saponin has been shown to have a significant anabolic effect on bone components in the femoral tissues of rats [184].

Ovarian hormone deficiency at menopause stimulates bone loss. Ovariectomy (OVX) causes a lack of estrogen, and the hormone deficiency induces osteoporosis in humans. Bone weight, bone mineral density, and bone mineral content were reduced in OVX rats [185]. Prolonged intake of fermented soybean diets with supplementation of isoflavone and saponin has been demonstrated to prevent bone loss in OVX rats [185], indicating that OVX-induced bone loss is prevented after prolonged intake of dietary isoflavone and saponin supplementation.

Fermented soybeans are food sources that largely contain genistein. The effect of experimental diets using fermented soybeans containing genistein on OVX-induced bone loss has also been demonstrated [185]. The experimental diets containing 44.6 to 92.4 mg of isoflavones (including genistein, genistein, daidzein, and daidzein) per 100 g of diet was fed to OVX rats for 3 months. OVX caused a significant reduction in the dry weight, mineral density, calcium content, and alkaline phosphatase activity in the femoral tissues [185]. These reductions were prevented after feeding a *natto* diet [185]. Thus, prolonged intake of dietary *natto* supplemented with isoflavone has preventive effects on OVX-induced bone loss, suggesting that it may have a role in the prevention of osteoporosis.

The effect of a standardized soy extract (SSE, Soyselect) in the OVX rat model of menopause has also been reported [186]. OVX rats were orally treated for 6 weeks with the soy extract (50 or 100 mg/kg/day), vehicle (distilled water), or 17β-estradiol (0.5 mg/kg/day) [186]. The SSE produced a bone-sparing effect associated with a slowing down in the increased bone turnover observed after OVX (as indicated by measurements of serum osteocalcin levels and excretion ratio of deoxypyridinoline) [186]. Remarkably, organ weight data and histopathologic analysis did not show any stimulatory activity of the SSE on the uterus [186]. Immunohistochemical analysis showed a significant down-regulation of estrogen receptor-α in uterine epithelium after 17β-estradiol treatment, but not after treatment with the SSE [186]. After treatment with 17β-estradiol, estrogen receptor-β expression was not modulated in the stroma or epithelium, whereas the SSE induced an up-regulation of estrogen receptor-β stromal expression [186]. Collectively, these findings suggest that the lack of stimulatory activity on the uterine epithelium using soy treatment could be due to a negligible stimulatory activity on estrogen receptor-α and/or to the enhanced expression observed in stromal estrogen receptor-β, the latter being considered as a negative modulator of estrogen receptor-α-mediated uterine proliferation. Uterine epithelial progesterone receptor was down-regulated by 17β-estradiol, but not the SSE, as compared with that in OVX rats [186]. The minor increase in lipid levels induced by OVX was not affected by SSE administration [186]. Thus, it has been demonstrated that the tested extract has an interesting profile of tissue-specific response, in that it is efficacious in preventing experimental osteoporosis without causing stimulation in uterus at doses that are effective in bone.

Preventive Effect of Dietary Soybean Genistein on Osteoporosis in Human Subjects

Twelve volunteers (six men and six women) were received *nijiru* twice a day for 60 days at a dose of 1500 mg (6 tablets) per day [187]. The serum γ-carboxylated osteocalcin concentration, which is a marker of osteoblastic bone formation, has been shown to significantly increase about 2-fold that in the control group after the intake of *nijiru* in both men and women to [187]. The intake of isoflavone- and saponin-containing *nijiru* stimulated the γ-carboxylation of osteocalcin, which plays an important role in osteoblastic bone formation and mineralization, in healthy individuals [187]. The dietary intake of foods including genistein may have a role in prevention of osteoporosis in human subjects.

The change in circulating biochemical markers of bone metabolism in aged individuals with the intake of fermented soybean (*natto*), which was made from isoflavone-rich soybean, has been examined [188]. Sixty-three volunteers (31 men and 32 women) were divided into four groups of 15 or 16 male volunteers and 16 or 16 female volunteers, and each group was sequentially given *natto* (40 g pack) containing once a day for 4 or 8 weeks as follows: either regular natto with naturally occuring isoflavone 35.0 mg and calcium 51.4 mg or supplemented *natto* containing isoflavone 35.0 mg and calcium 60.0 mg.

As serum bone markers, bone-specific alkaline phosphatase, γ-carboxylated osteocalcin, bone tartrate-resistant acid phosphatase (TRACP), and N-telopeptide of type I collagen were assayed. The intake of regular *natto* for 4 or 8 weeks in men or women persons caused a significant increase in γ-carboxylated osteocalcin, a marker of bone formation, and a significant decrease in serum bone N-teleopeptide of type I collagen, a marker of bone resorption, as compared with the value before intake [188]. Moreover, the intake of *natto* for 8 weeks in men or women caused a significant increase in serum bone-specific alkaline phosphatase activity and γ-carboxylated osteocalcin concentration and a significant decrease in serum bone TRACP activity and N-telopeptide of type I collagen, as compared with the values with intake of regular *natto* [188]. This study suggests that the intake of regular *natto* with isoflavone-rich soybean has stimulatory effects on bone formation and suppressive effects on bone resorption in aged individuals.

Thus, prolonged intake of dietary genistein may be usefulness for bone health, prevention and treatment of bone loss with aging and various pathophysiolocal states.

Conclusion

Bone homeostasis, which is regulated through osteoblastic cells and osteoclastic cells in bone tissues, is disordered with aging and pathophysiologic state including menopause. This leads to bone loss, which may be due to decreased osteoblastic bone formation and increased osteoclastic bone resorption. Bone loss induces bone fracture, which is public problem. Functional food factors may help to prevent bone loss with aging. This may be important in maintaining bone health in long life. Genistein, which are largely contained in soybean, has been demonstrated to stimulate osteoblastic bone formation and to suppress osteoclastic bone resorption, suggesting a new molecular mechanism in the regulation of bone homeostasis. Genistein has been shown to have stimulatory effects on osteoblastic bone formation and suppressive effects on osteoclastic bone resorption. Genistein stimulates protein synthesis and gene expression of proteins which are involved in osteobalstic cell and osteoclastic cell functions. Genistein induces apoptosis of mature osteoclasts. Fermented soybeans (*natto*) are good food sources that largely contain genistein. Dietary fermented soybean intake has a great effect in the prevention and treatment of bone loss in animal models and humans. Moreover, prevention of bone fracture with dietary fermented soybean intake is supported through epidemiologic investigation in Japan. Dietary soybean genistein as a biomedical food factor may be useful in the prevention and treatment of osteoporosis induced by various pathophysiologic states.

Chapter 4

Synergistic Effect of Zinc and Genistein on Osteoporosis Treatment

As described in Chapter 2 and 3, zinc, an essential trace element, and genistein, an isoflavone which are largely contained in soybeans, has been shown to have stimulatory effects on osteoblastic bone formation and suppressive effects on osteoclastic bone resorption, thereby increasing bone mass. These factors are based on the effects on protein synthesis and gene expression of various proteins, which are related to osteblastic bone formation and osteoclastic bone resorption. Functional food factors, which are nutrients, may have a potent effect to delay degenerative bone disorders such as osteoporosis. The authors had an idea that the combination of these factors may have synergistic effects on bone. The combination of zinc and genistein was found to have a synergistic effect on osteogenesis, and such combination was useful to prevent and treat bone loss induced in various pathophysiological states [189]. Moreover, the supplemental intake of ingredients with the combination of zinc and genistein has been shown to have potent effects on osteoporosis in human subjects. The combination of functional food factors may play a role in the prevention and treatment of osteoporosis. This knowledge may be important in the prevention of bone loss with age and treatment of osteoporosis of postmenopausal women.

Synergistic Effects of Zinc and Genistein on Bone *In Vivo*

The effect of zinc sulfate (5.5 mg/kg body weight) on DNA and calcium contents in the femoral tissues has been found to synergisctically enhance after simultaneous administration of genistein (100 μg/kg body weight) *in vivo* [189-192]. Oral administration of genistein (100 and 300 μg/kg) or zinc sulfate (1 and 5 mg Zn/kg) to female rats for 3 days caused a significant increase in alkaline phosphatase activity, DNA, and calcium content in the femoral-metaphyseal tissues *in vivo* [190]. The synergistic effect was seen in case of genistein (100 and 300 μg/kg) plus zinc (5 mg/kg) [190]. The combination of zinc and genistein may be a useful tool in the prevention and therapy of osteoporosis.

Zinc and Genistein Synergistically Stimulates Osteoblastogenesis

The cellular and molecular mechanisms by which zinc enhances anabolic effect of genistein on bone components have been investigated. The combination of zinc (10^{-5} or 10^{-4} M) and genistein (10^{-6} or 10^{-5} M) was found to have additive and synergistic effects on protein content in osteoblastic MC3T3-E1 cells *in vitro* [193]. This effect may involve the activation of aminoacyl-tRNA synthase by zinc and genistein, since these factors can increase the enzyme activity in the cytosol of osteoblastic cells *in vitro* [193].

Alkaline phosphatase is an enzyme marker of osteoblasts and the enzyme participates in bone mineralization [159]. α1 (I) collagen is a matrix protein that is related to bone formation and mineralization in osteoblast lineage cells [159]. Osteocalcin is a bone matrix protein containing γ_2-carboxyglutamin acid, which is synthesized in osteoblasts and is the protein involved in mineralization [159]. The expression of alkaline phosphatase, α1 (I) collagen, and osteocalcin mRNAs in osteoblastic cells was synergistically enhanced after culture with combination of zinc (10^{-5} or 10^{-4} M) and genistein (10^{-6} or 10^{-5} M) as compared to effects of each factor [193]. This finding demonstrates that the combination of zinc and genistein has a synergistic effect on gene expression in osteoblastic cells.

The effect of the combination of zinc (10^{-4} M) and genistein (10^{-5} M) on the gene expression in osteoblastic cells was completely prevented in the presence of cycloheximide, an inhibitor of protein synthesis, and DRB, an inhibitor of transcriptional activity [193]. This suggests that the combination of genistein and zinc stimulates the transcriptional process in osteoblastic cells. Zinc or genistein has a stimulatory effect on protein synthesis at the transcriptional process. Presumably, the combination of zinc and genistein stimulates both transcriptional and translational activities in osteoblastic cells. Each factor activates aminoacyl-tRNA synthetase at the transcriptional process in osteoblastic cells. It has been speculated that zinc or genistein has an effect on the binding of transcriptional factor(s), which is synthesized through the translational process, to the nuclear DNA in osteoblastic cells.

Culture with zinc (10^{-4} M) and genistein (10^{-5} M) has a stimulatory effect on mineralization in osteoblastic cells [193]. The combination of zinc and genistein synergistically enhanced mineralization in osteoblastic cells. This finding supportes the view that the combination of zinc and genistein can effectively enhance bone mineralization, thereby increasing bone mass [193].

Zinc and Genistein Synergistically Inhibits Osteoclastogenesis

The combination of zinc (10^{-5} M) and genistein (10^{-6} M) has been shown to have a potent-suppressive effect on osteoclastogenesis as compared with effects of each factor [194]. Culture with PTH markedly stimulated the formation of osteoclast-like cells in mouse marrow culture [194]. This stimulation was significantly inhibited in the presence of zinc or genistein. The additive effects were seen with the combination of zinc (10^{-5} M) plus genistein (10^{-6} M) or zinc (10^{-4} M) plus genistein (10^{-5} M). The effects of two combinations with different concentrations were saturated with used concentration [194].

The combination of zinc (10^{-5} M) and genistein (10^{-6} M) has also been shown to have a potent-suppressive effect on osteoclastic cells, which are generated in mouse marrow culture with macropharge-colony stimulating factor (M-CSF) and RANKL *in vitro* [194]. The number of mature osteoclastic cells was synergistically decreased after culture of zinc (10^{-5} M) plus genistein (10^{-6} M) as compared with the effects of each factor. The combination of zinc and genistein had a potent-suppressive effect on mature osteoclastic cells [194]. This effect was remarkable in the presence of M-CSF and RANKL, although it was also seen in the absence of M-CSF and RANKL [194]. The combination of zinc and genistein may have suppressive effects on RANKL signaling-dependent pathways in osteoclastic cells.

Culture with zinc (10^{-5} M) and genistein (10^{-6} M) caused a synergistic increase in DNA fragmentation in osteoclastic cells [194], indicating that both factors stimulate apoptotic cell death. In addition, zinc plus genistein-induced cell death was significantly prevented in the presence of caspase-3 inhibitor [194]. However, this effect was partial. Presumably, the stimulation of apoptotic cell death with the combination of zinc and genistein is partly mediated through the activation of caspase-3, and also other mechanisms may particapate in apoptotic cell death.

Zinc (10^{-5} M) increases the expression of caspase-3 mRNA in osteoclastic cells cultured with or without M-CSF and RANKL [194]. This effect was significantly enhanced with the combination of genistein (10^{-6} M). However, genistein did not have effect in the presence of M-CSF and RANKL, supporting the view that the combination of zinc and genistein has a potent-stimulatory effect on apoptotic cell death, which is partly mediated through caspase-3 in osteoclastic cells [194].

The stimulatory effects with combination of zinc (10^{-5} M) and genistein (10^{-6} M) on caspase-3 mRNA expression was completely inhibited after culture with cycloheximide, an inhibitor of protein synthesis, or DRB, an inhibitor of transcriptional activity, in osteoclastic cells with or without M-CSF and RANKL [194]. This finding suggests that the effects with combination of zinc and genistein on caspase-3 mRNA expression are involved in protein synthesis and transcription activation in osteoclastic cells. Moreover, zinc or genistein has been demonstrated to have stimulatory effects on protein synthesis due to activating aminoacyl-tRNA synthetase, a rate-limiting enzyme in protein synthesis, in osteoblastic cells.

The activation of TRACP or cathepsin K plays a role in the promotion of osteoclastic bone resorption by stimulating the decomposition of bone matrix [7, 8, 78]. The expression of TRACP mRNA was significantly decreased in the presence of genistein plus zinc in osteoclastic cells cultured with M-CSF and RANKL for 72 hours, although the method with reverse transcriprtion-polymerase chain reaction (RT-PCR) is qualitative/semi-quantitative determination. Zinc (10^{-5} M) or genistein (10^{-6} M) alone did not have a significant effect on TRACP mRNA in osteoclastic cells [194].

Culture with zinc or genistein for 72 hours was also found to induce a significant decrease in cathepsin K mRNA expression in osteoclastic cells cultured in the presence or absence of M-CSF and RANKL [194]. The combination of zinc and genistein had a potent suppressive effect on cathepsin K mRNA expression as compared with effects of each factor [194].

These findings demonstrate that the combination of zinc (10^{-5} M) and genistein (10^{-6} M) has synergistic-suppressive effects on the activity of TRACP or cathepsin K in osteoclastic cells which are activated through RANKL signaling. The combination of zinc and genistein has a potent suppressive effect on bone-resorbing activity.

RANK activation by binding of RANKL on preosteoclasts stimulates the NF-κB signaling, propbably through association with TRAF-6 in osteoclasts. RANKL signaling targets include mitogen-activated protein kinases (MAPKs), NF-κB, and nuclear factor of activated T cells c1 (NFATc1) in osteoclast differentiation [195].

Culture with combination of zinc (10^{-5} M) and genistein (10^{-6} M) did not cause a significant change in NF-κB mRNA expression in osteoclastic cells in the presence or absence of M-CSF and RANKL [193]. NFATc1 mRNA expression was significantly increased after culture with the combination of zinc (10^{-5} M) and genistein (10^{-6} M) in osteoclastic cells cultured in the presence of M-CSF and RANKL [193]. Zinc and genistein may affect on the gene expression of NFATc1 that is a target protein of RANKL signaling in osteoclastic cells. The decrease in NFATc1 expression with combination of zinc and genistein may be important in the revelation of synergistic-suppressive effects on osteoclastogenesis and osteoclastic cell function.

In conclusion, the combination of zinc and genistein has been found to have additive or synergistic effects on the suppressions of PTH-induced osteoclastogenesis, mature osteoclastic cell death, and bone resorption-related gene expression in osteoclastic cells in presence of M-CSF and RANKL.

The mechanism by which the combination of zinc and genistein has additive or synergistic effects on osteogenesis is shown in Figure 9.

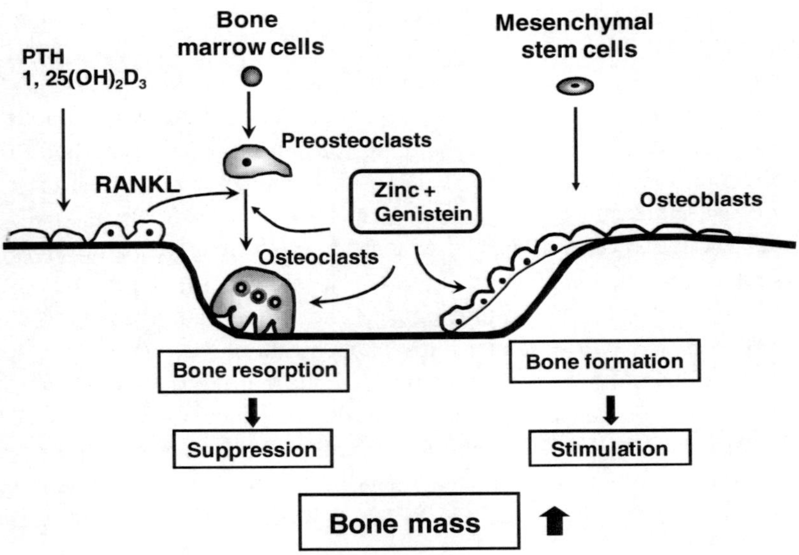

Figure 9. The combination of zinc and genistein has synergistic effects on stimulation of osteoblastic bone formation and suppression of osteoclastic bone resorption, thereby increasing bone mass. These factors stimulate cell differentiation, cell proliferation and mineralization in osteoblasts and suppress osteoclastogenesis that is induced by various bone-resorbing factors in bone marrow culture. In addition, the combination of these factors regulates protein synthesis and gene expression of various proteins, which are related to finctions of osteoblasts and osteoclasts.

Supplemental Intake of Zinc and Genistein Has Potent-preventive Effects on Bone Loss

As mentioned above, the combination of zinc and genistein has been demonstrated to have synergistic effects on the stimulation of osteoblastic bone formation [193] and the suppression of osteoclastic bone resorption [194], thereby increasing bone mass. The combination of dietary zinc and genistein may have a potent role in the prevention of bone loss with various pathophysiologic states.

Fermented soybeans are a good food source, which largely contain both zinc and genistein. The effects of experimental diets with fermented soybeans containing zinc and genistein on OVX-induced bone loss has been demonstrated [196]. The experimental diets containing 2.1 to 9.7 mg of zinc per 100 g of diet and 44.6 to 92.4 mg of isoflavones (including genistein, genistin, daidzein and daidzin) per 100 g of diet was fed to OVX rats for 3 months. OVX caused a significant reduction in the dry weight, mineral density, calcium content, zinc content, and alkaline phosphatase activity in femoral tissues [196]. These reductions were prevented after feeding a *natto* diet. This prevention was significantly enhanced in OVX rats fed a *natto* diet supplemented with zinc and isoflavone. Prolonged intake of dietary *natto* supplemented with zinc and isoflavone has preventive effects on OVX-induced bone loss, suggesting that it may have a role in the prevention of osteoporosis.

The change in circulating biochemical markers of bone metabolism in aged individuals with the intake of fermented soybean (*natto*), which was made from isoflavone-rich soybean, supplemented with zinc has been examined [197]. Sixty-three volunteers (31 men and 32 women) were divided into four groups of 15 or 16 male volunteers and 16 or 16 female volunteers, and each group was sequentially given *natto* (40 g pack) containing two different levels of zinc once a day for 4 or 8 weeks as follows: either regular natto with naturally occuring isoflavone 35.0 mg, zinc 0.8 mg and calcium 51.4 mg or supplemented *natto* containing isoflavone 35.0 mg, zinc 3.6 mg, and calcium 60.0 mg.

As serum bone markers, bone-specific alkaline phosphatase, γ-carboxylated osteocalcin, bone tartrate-resistant acid phosphatase (TRACP), and N-telopeptide of type I collagen were used to analysis of effects. Intake of regular *natto* for 4 or 8 weeks in men or women persons caused a significant increase in γ-carboxylated osteocalcin, a marker of bone formation, and a significant decrease in serum bone N-teleopeptide of type I collagen, a marker of bone resorption, as compared with the value before intake [197]. Moreover, the intake of zinc-supplemented *natto* for 8 weeks in men or women caused a significant increase in serum bone-specific alkaline phosphatase activity and γ-carboxylated osteocalcin concentration and a significant decrease in serum bone TRACP activity and N-telopeptide of type I collagen, as compared with the values with the intake of regular *natto* [197].

This study suggests that the intake of regular *natto* with isoflavone-rich soybean has a stimulatory effect on bone formation and an inhibitory effect on bone resorption in aged individuals, and that this effect is significantly enhanced by supplementation with zinc.

Zinc or genistein has been shown to have stimulatory effects on osteoblastic bone formation and suppressive effects on osteoclastic bone resorption. The potent-preventive effects of dietary isoflavone (richly including genistein) with zinc supplementation may result from synergistic effects with zinc and genistein on osteoblasts and osteoclasts in the bone tissues of aged individuals. Prolonged intake of dietary genistein with zinc supplementation may be useful in the prevention of bone loss with aging and in treatment of osteoporosis with various pathophysiolocal states.

Conclusion

Bone loss may be due to decreased osteoblastic bone formation and increased osteoclastic bone resorption. Functional food factors are needed to prevent bone loss with increasing age. Zinc, an essential trace element, and genistein, which is largely contained in soybean, has potential-stimulatory effects on osteoblastic bone formation and suppressive effects on osteoclastic bone resorption, thereby increasing bone mass. These factors regulate the gene expression of many proteins, which are related to the functions of osteoblastic and osteoclastic cells.

The combination with zinc and genistein has been found to have synergistic effects in the prevention and treatment of bone loss induced in ovariectomized rats, which are an animal model of osteoporosis, due to stimulating osteoblastic bone formation and inhibiting osteoclastic bone resorption. Moreover, these combinations have been demonstrated to have synergistic-anabolic effects on bone in humans. However, the author could not find out synergistic effects or additive effects with combination of over three factors (compounds) on bone mass thus far. In addition, the combination either genistein, menaquinon-7 (Chapter 5), or β-cryptoxanthin (Chapter 6) had additive effects, but not synergistic effects, on bone.

Zinc was essential factor which has synerigistic effects with combination of functional food factors on bone. The supplemental intake with combination of zinc and genistein may play an important role in the prevention and treatment of bone loss with various pathophysiologic states. Currently, the author cannot provide information on ethnic, gender and geographic variation in osteoporosis and how this could impact recommendations for dietary and supplemental intakes of dietary combination of zinc and other factors. However, it has been shown that dietary intake of fermented soybeans (*natto*), which richly contain zinc and genistein, can prevent bone fracture with epidemiologic investigation in Japan, although further investigation is needed in the world levels.

Drugs, which are clinically used in the treatment of osteoporosis, are mainly based on the action of osteoclastic bone resorption. Clinical compound that stimulates bone formation is very few.

As described in this chapter, zinc or genistein has a stimulatory effect on bone formation, and their combination has a synergistic-anabolic effect on bone. The combination of zinc and genistein may be a potential-useful tool in therapy of osteoporosis. This may be used as a new drug (biomedical food product), which stimulates osteoblastic bone formation and suppresses osteoclastic bone resorption, thereby increasing bone mass.

Chapter 5

Role of Fermented Soybean Menaquinone-7 (Vitamin K_2) in Osteoporosis Treatment

Vitamin K is a fat-soluble vitamin that was originally identified as an essential factor for blood coagulation. Vitamin K is co-factor of γ-carboxylase that glutamate residues of osteocalcin, a protein synthesized by osteoblasts, are converted into γ-carboxyglutamate (Gla). Since its discovery in the 1930s, the importance of vitamin K in physiological processes other than blood coagulation has become increasingly clear. Vitamin K has been shown to have multiple functions. Recent advances in the discovery of new functions for vitamin K-dependent proteins have clarified physiological roles of vitamin K in bone mineralization, arterial calcification, apoptosis, phagocytosis, growth control, chemotaxis, and signal transduction [198].

There are three types of vitamin K: vitamin K_1 (phylloquinone), vitamin K_2 (menaquinone), and vitamin K_3 (menadione). Vitamin K_1 is a sole compound, but vitamin K_2 is a series of vitamers with multiisoprene units (one to four) at the 3-position of the naphthoquinone, which are classified according to the length of their aliphatic side chain and are designated as MK-n, where n stands for the number of isoprenoid residues in that chain. Chemical structure of vitamin K is shown in Figure 10.

Several reports have found the effects of vitamin K on bone metabolism [199-202]. Like vitamin K_1 (phylloquinone), vitamin K_2 (menaquinone-4; MK-4), with four isoprene units, not only enhances mineralization but also increases the amount of osteocalcin in cultured human osteoblasts [199]. MK-4 is essential for the γ-carboxylation of osteocalcin, a bone matrix protein containing γ_2-carboxyglutamic acids, which are synthesized in osteoblasts of bone tissues [200, 201]. Noncarboxylated osteocalcin cannot bind to hydroxyapatite in mineralized tissues [202]. MK-4 has been shown to inhibit bone resorption, which may be related to its side chain, and it can inhibit bone loss in ovariectomized rats [203].

Natural menaquinone-7 (MK-7; vitamin K_2) with seven isoprene units is very abundant in fermented soybean, although it is only slight in other foods. It has been shown that serum MK-7 concentration in women living in Tokyo, where fermented soybean is consumed, is about ten times higher than that of those living in Europe [204]. These differences may result from the intake of fermented soybean (*natto*). An appropriate amount of MK-7 intake through diet may be significant in preventing age-related bone loss.

The author *et al.* found that MK-7 has an anabolic effect on bone calcification in rat femoral tissues *in vitro* [205]. This was the first time finding. MK-7 can directly stimulate calcification in the femoral-metaphyseal tissues obtained from normal and aged rats *in vitro* [206]. Action of MK-7 on bone calcification has been shown to have the same effect as MK-4. MK-7 has partially been converted to MK-4 in the body. MK-7 may have an important role in the prevention of osteoporosis with aging. Intestinal absorption of vitamin K from diet gradually declines with advancing age. Consequently, vitamin K deficiency may occur with aging. Vitamin K_2 may be important in bone healthy [207, 208].

Aging induces a reduction in bone mass by decrease in osteoblactic bone formation and increase in osteoclastic bone resorption. Malnutrition or undernutrition is often observed in the elderly, and it appears to be more intense in patients with hip fracture than in the general aging population [2]. The deficiency in both micronutrients and macronutrients appears to be strongly implicated in the pathogenesis and the consequences of hip fracture in the osteoporotic elderly. Nutritional factors have been shown to be important in preventing bone loss with increasing age [209-210]. Intestinal absorption of vitamin K from diet gradually declines with advancing age. Consequently, vitamin K deficiency may occur with aging. Dietary vitamin K_2 may be important in the prevention of osteoporosis with aging.

This chapter introduces findings concerning the role of vitamin K_2 (menaquinone-7; MK-7), which enhances γ-carboxylation of bone glutamic acid residues of osteocalcin, in the regulation of bone homeostasis *in vitro* and its preventive effect on osteoporosis in animals *in vivo* and human subjects.

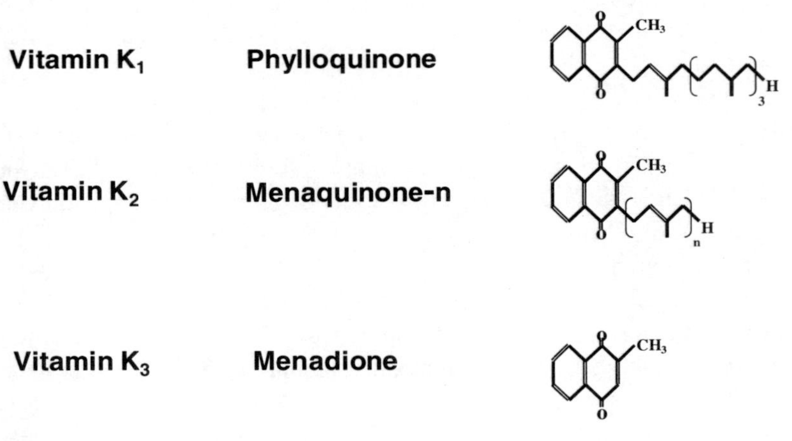

Figure 10. Chemical structure of Vitamin K.

Function of Vitamin K

Vitamin K is an essential cofactor for the post-translational carboxylation of certain protein-bound glutamate residues of osteocalcin, a synthesized by osteobalsts, which are converted into gamma-carboxy glutamate (Gla) by γ-carboxylase [213, 214]. These Gla residues form calcium-binding sites that are essential for the activity of the proteins. During gamma-glutamate carboxylation, vitamin K is oxidized into its epoxide form (KO), which is reconverted to vitamin K quinone (K) by the enzyme vitamin K epoxide reductase (VKOR). Derivatives of 4-hydroxycoumarin (including warfarin and acenocoumarol) specifically inhibit VKOR, thus preventing the recycling of vitamin K [215]. In this carboxylation process, glutamate residues are converted into γ-carboxyglutamate (Gla) [214]. These Gla residues have a high affinity for calcium, which is an essential property of all Gla proteins.

Well-known Gla-containing proteins are the blood coagulation factors II, VII, IX, and X, which are all synthesized in the liver [214]. Gla proteins not related with blood clotting are osteocalcin (synthesized in bone) and matrix Gla protein (primarily synthesized in cartilage and in the vessel wall) [213, 214]. The only unequivocal deficiency outcome is a bleeding syndrome caused by an inability to synthesize active coagulation factors II, VII, IX, and X.

In recent years, there is growing evidence for the roles of vitamin K in bone and vascular health [215-217]. Vitamin K_2 activates osteoblasts to enhance mineralization *in vitro*. Clinically, vitamin K_2 maintains lumbar bone mineral density (BMD) and prevents osteoporotic fractures in patients with osteoporosis.

Vitamin K and Bone Metabolism

Osteocalcin is one of the bone matrix proteins; it is vitamin K dependent, and is synthesized in osteoblasts in the bone tissues. The fraction newly synthesized by osteoblasts is released into circulation. For this reason, the circulating levels of osteocalcin are considered sensitive markers of bone formation [218, 219]. Among the osteocalcins, fully carboxylated osteocalcin has a high affinity to calcium and/or hydroxyapataite, and may play an important role in maintaining bone mineral density (BMD) and reducing the incidence of fractures through incremental bone formation [219].

Several studies in adults suggest a beneficial role for vitamin K in bone mineral metabolism and bone fracture prevention [220]. A well-recognized concept is a vital role of vitamin K. A poor vitamin K status will lead to production of undercarboxylated (inactive) osteocalcin (unOC) [221]. In the healthy adult population, osteocalcin is carboxylated to a variable extent, suggesting that the intake dietary vitamin K is often insufficient for all osteocalcin carboxylation. In postmenopausal women, a clear association between elevated unOC and increased fracture risk is found [220].

Patients with hip fracture have significantly lower vitamin K_1 levels than those in the controls [208]. Significantly lower levels of vitamin K_1 and vitamin K_2 are found in the serum obtained from elderly patients within a few hours after a hip fracture [222]. A low vitamin K_1 intake is one of the risk factors in hip fracture. Higher vitamin K_1 levels than the current recommendation for coagulation parameters may be required for carboxylation of osteocalcin [223]. The fractions of osteocalcin with a high affinity to hydroxyapatite are increased following vitamin K_1 administration, accompanied by a reduction in urinary calcium excretion [224]. A daily vitamin K_1 supplement of 80 μg seems to be necessary to reach a premenopausal carboxylated osteocalcin/total osteocalcin ratio [225]. These findings suggest that vitamin K deficiency may be responsible for reduced carboxylation of osteocalcin and may be one of the risk factors in low bone mass resulting in fragility fractures. The administration of vitamin K may ameliorate undercarboxylation of osteocalcin in the elderly with osteoporosis [219]. Intake of dietary vitamin K is potentially beneficial for bone.

Dietary Vitamin K

In food. the most important K vitamins are K_1 (notably found in green vegetables and some plant oils) and the long-chain menaquinones (MK) including MK-7, MK-8, and MK-9 (present in fermented foods, notably cheese and *natto*). *Natto* consists of fermented soybeans and is popular food in Japan, but because of its strong taste it is not well appreciated elsewhere. It is the richest dietary source of vitamin K presently known, almost all of which occurs in the form of MK-7.

In food supplements, 3 forms of vitamin K may be found: MK-4 (prepared by organ synthesis and almost exclusively used in Japan), vitamin K_1 (also synthetic and predominant form used in the rest of the world), and MK-7 (a natural form prepared by extraction of *natto* food). Since the molecular structures of vitamin K_1 and MK-4 are comparable (both contain 4 isoprenoid residues, 3 of which are saturated in vitamin K_1 but contain a double bond in MK-4), their physico-chemical characteristics are closely similar.

The higher menaquinones including MK-7 are much more hydrophobic, however, and *in vivo* they are handled differently: they have longer half-life times [216], and in the circulation they are incorporated into low-density lipoproteins [217]. Vitamin K_1 is by far the most common form of vitamin K in commercially available supplements, but because of the health claims for the regular consumption of *natto*. MK-7 in the form of a *natto* extract is rapidly gaining interest. Whereas supplements containing vitamin K_1 have been commercially available for many years, MK-7 has central the market only recently.

An adult daily intake of about 100 μg of vitamin K_1 is recommended for the maintenance of hemostasis [213]. Traditional coagulation tests for assessing vitamin K status are nonspecific and insensitive. Better tests include measurements of circulating vitamin K and inactive proteins such as undercarboxylated forms of factor II and osteocalcin to assess tissue and functional status, respectively.

The common risk factors for vitamin K deficiency in the hospitalized patient include inadequate dietary intakes, malabsorption syndromes (especially owing to chlestatic liver diseas), antibiotic therapy, and renal insufficiency [213]. The pregnant women and their newborns present a special risk category because of poor placental transport and low concentrations of vitamin K in breast milk [213]. Since 2000, the Food and Drug Administration has mandated that adult parenteral preparations should provide a supplemental amount of 150 μg vitamin K_1 per day in addition to that present naturally, in variable amounts, in the lipid emulsion [213]. Although this supplemental daily amount is probably beneficial in preventing vitamin K deficiency, it may be excessive for patients taking vitamin K antagonists, such as warfarin, and jeopardize their anticoagulation control. Natural forms of vitamin K have no proven toxicity.

Menaquinone-7 and Bone Homeostasis

The author *et al.* firstly found that menaquinone-7 (MK-7), which was isolated from *natto*, has anabolic effects on bone calcification in rat femoral tissues *in vitro* [205]. MK-7 can directly stimulate calcification in the femoral tissues obtained from normal and aged rats *in vitro* [205]. The action of MK-7 on bone calcification has been shown to have the same effect as MK-4. MK-7 has partially been converted to MK-4 in the body. MK-7 may have an important role in the prevention of osteoporosis.

MK-7 Stimulates Osteoblastic Bone Formation

MK-7 has been found to have a stimulatory effect on calcification in the femoral tissues obtained from normal young rats *in vitro* [205]. Culture with MK-7 (10^{-6} or 10^{-5} M) caused a significant increase in biochemical components (alkaline phosphatase acitivy, DNA and calcium contents) in the femoral-diaphyseal (cortical bone) and -metaphyseal (trabecular bone) tissues obtained from aged rats *in vitro* [206]. The effect of MK-7 was significantly enhanced in the presence of genistein (10^{-6} or 10^{-5} M), suggesting that the mode of action of MK-7 differs from that of genistein [206]. The effect of MK-7 in increasing bone components in the femoral tissues was completely abolished in the presence of cycloheximide, an inhibitory of protein syntheasis *in vitro* [206]. Thus, MK-7 has stimulatory effects on bone formation in the femoral tissues of elderly female rats *in vitro*.

Osteoblastic MC3T3-E1 cells with subconfluency were cultured for 24 hours in a serum-free medium containing MK-7 (10^{-7} - 10^{-5} M) [226]. Culture with MK-7 (10^{-6} or 10^{-5} M) caused a significant increase in alkaline phosphatase activity, protein and DNA contents in osteoblastic cells [226]. The effect of MK-7 on cellular alkaline phosphatase activity and osteocalcin concentration was completely depressed in the presence of cycloheximide. MK-7 has a stimulatory effect on osteoblastic bone formation due to increasing protein synthesis including osteocalcin.

MK-7 Suppresses Osteocalstic Bone Resorption

MK-7 has been shown to have suppressive effects on oteoclastic bone resoption in *vitro* [227]. Culture with parathyroid hormone (PTH) and prostaglandin E_2 (PGE_2), which are bone-resorbing factors, caused a significant decrease in calcium content in the femoral-metaphyseal tissues obtained from young and aged rats *in vitro* [227]. Bone-resorbing factor-induced decrease in metaphyseal calcium content was completely prevented after culture with MK-7 (10^{-7} - 10^{-5} M), indicating that MK-7 has inhibitory effects on bone resorption in bone tissue culture [227].

In addition, MK-7 (10^{-7} - 10^{-5} M) completely suppressed PTH- or PGE_2-induced increase in medium glucose consumption and lactic acid production by bone tissues *in vitro* [227]. The suppressive effects of MK-7 on bone resorption may partly result from inhibition of PTH- or PGE_2-stimulated medium glucose consumption and lactic acid production by the bone tissues [227]. PTH stimulates extracellular release of lactic acid from osteoclastic cells. PTH-induced increase in lactic acid production may result from consumption of glucose by osteoclastic cells [227]. This acid production may have an importance as cellular mechanism of bone resorption.

Osteoclast-like cells are formed from bone marrow cells in the presence of bone-resorbing factors (PTH or PGE_2) [227]. PTH- or PGE_2-induced increase in osteoclast-like cell formation was significantly inhibited by MK-7 ($10^{-8} – 10^{-5}$ M) [227]. MK-7 had more potent-suppressive effects at later stage of the differentiation of marrow cells. Osteoclast-like cell formation was stimulated when dibutyryl cyclic AMP (DcAMP) or phorbol 12-myristate 13-acetate (PMA), an activator of protein kinase C, was added into culture medium. MK-7 significantly inhibited effect of PMA on osteoclast-like cell formation, although it did not have inhibitory effects on DcAMP-induced increase in osteoclast-like cell formation. These observations suggest that suppressive effects of MK-7 are partly involved in protein kinase C signaling [227].

The effect of MK-7 on mature osteoclasts isolated from rat femoral tissues has been examined [227]. Culture with MK-7 (10^{-6} or 10^{-5} M) caused a significant decrease in the number of mature osteoclasts. This decrease was also seen in the presence of calcitonin, DcAMP or calcium chloride [227]. The effect of MK-7 in decreasing the number of osteoclasts was not further enhanced in the presence of calcitonin, DcAMP, or calcium chloride, and it was completely abolished in the presence of dibucaine or staurosporine, which are inhibitors of Ca^{2+}-dependent protein kinases. Suppressive effects of MK-7 on osteoclasts may be partly mediated through the pathways of Ca^{2+}- and cyclic AMP-dependent signalings [227].

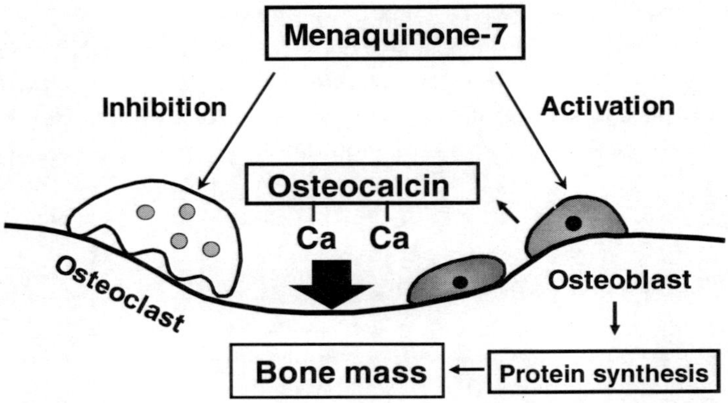

Figure 11. Menaquinone-7 (MK-7) stimulates osteoblastogenesis and suppresses osteoclastogenesis, thereby increasing bone mass. MK-7 stimulates protein synthesis including osteocalcin and other protein molecules in osteoblastic cells. In addition, MK-7 regulates gene expressions of proteins, which are reraleted to ostebalstic and osteoclastic cell functions.

Mechanism of MK-7 Action in Bone Homeostasis

MK-7 has been shown to stimulate osteoblastic bone formation and osteoclastic bone resorption, thereby increasing bone mass, as shown in Figure 11. MK-7 may activate γ-carboxylase that glutamate residues of osteocalcin are converted into γ-carboxyglutamate in osteoblastic cells. MK-7 stimulates protein synthesis including osteocalcin in osteoblastic cells [226].

The activation of NF-κB signal transduction pathway is essential for osteoclast formation and resorption. By contrast, NF-κB signaling potently antagonizes osteoblast differentiation and function. Vitamin K_2 action on osteoblast and osteoclast formation and activity is accomplished by downregulating basal and cytokine-induced NF-κB activation, by increasing IκB mRNA, in a γ-carboxylation-independent manner [228]. Vitamin K_2 further prevented repression by TNF-α of Smad signaling induced by either TGF-β or BMP-2 [228]. Vitamin K_2 further antagonized receptor activator of NF-κB (RANK) ligand (RANKL)-induced NF-κB activation in osteoclast precursors [228]. These findings provide a novel mechanism to explain the dual pro-anabolic and anti-catabolic activities of vitamin K_2 as shown in Figure 12, and further support the concept that pharmacological modulation of NF-κB signal transduction may constitute an effective mechanism for ameliorating pathological bone loss and for promoting bone health [228]. Moreover, the suppressive effects of MK-7 on osteoclasts may be partly mediated through the pathway of Ca^{2+}- and cyclic AMP-dependent signalings [227].

Vitamin K_2 has also been shown to be a transcription regulator of bone-specific genes that act through steroid and xenobiotic receptors (SXRs) to promote expression of osteoblastic markers [229].

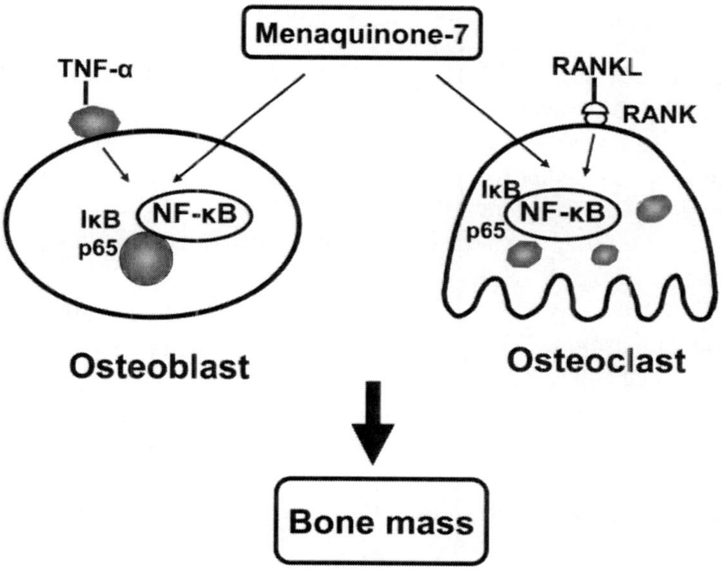

Figure 12. Menaquinone-7 (MK-7) stimulates osteoblastogenesis and suppresses osteoclastogenesis. As this signaling mechanism, it is important that MK-7 suppresses NF-κB signaling pathways in osteoblasts and osteoclasts. In addition, MK-7 stimulates protein synthesis including osteocalcin and other protein molecules in osteoblastic cells and regulates gene expressions of proteins, which are reraleted to functions in ostebalstic and osteoclastic cells.

Dietary MK-7 Intake Prevents Bone Loss

MK-7 increases bone mass due to stimulating osteoblastic bone formation and inhibiting osteoclastic bone resorption, suggesting that MK-7 has a preventive effect on osteoporosis. The preventive effects of dietary MK-7 on bone loss have been shown using ovariectomized (OVX) rats [230]. OVX rats were given experimental diets containing MK-4 (12 mg/100 g diet) or MK-7 (18.1 mg/100 g diet) for 24 days; MK-4 and MK-7 were equal in molar concentration [230]. This feeding caused remarkable increases in MK-4 and MK-7 concentrations in the serum and femur of OVX rats. OVX-induced decrease in the femoral dry weight and calcium content were prevented after feeding with dietary MK-4 or MK-7 [230].

In separate experiments, OVX rats were given experimental diets containing fermented soybeans (*natto*; including MK-7, 9.4 μg/100 g diet) with or without added MK-7 (37.6 μg/100 g diet) for 77 days [230]. Feeding produced a significant elevation of MK-4 and MK-7 concentrations in the serum of OVX rats. The decreases in the femoral dry weight and femoral calcium content induced by OVX were significantly prevented after feeding with diets containing natto with MK-7 added (37.6 μg/100 g diet) [230]. This effect was not seen with diets containing *natto* without MK-7 or both MK-7 and isoflavone [230]. The intake of dietary MK-7 has a preventive effect on bone loss caused by OVX. This effect may be partly contributed to MK-4 that is formed after degradation of MK-7 in body.

The effect of prolonged intake of dietary MK-7 on bone loss in OVX rats has also been shown [231]. OVX rats were given experimental diets containing fermented soybeans (including MK-7, 9.4 μg/100 g diet) with or without supplemental MK-7 (containing 14.1 or 18.8 μg/100 g diet) for 150 days [231]. Feeding produced a significant elevation of the MK-7 serum concentration of OVX rats [231]. Serum γ-carboxylated osteocalcin concentration was significantly decreased after OVX. This decrease was significantly prevented after the feeding of natto diets with supplemental MK-7 (18.8 μg/100 g diet) [231]. OVX caused a significant decrease in femoral dry weight, femoral calcium content, and mineral density. These decreases were significantly prevented after feeding with diets containing natto, which includes MK-7 (total, 18.8 μg/100 g diet) [231].

Co-relationship with dietary MK-7 intake and bone formation markers in OVX rats showed a good co-relationship [231].

Thus, prolonged intake of natto with MK-7 has been shown to have preventive effects on bone loss induced by OVX. Dietary MK-7 may be useful in the prevention of osteoporosis.

Anabolic Effects of mk-7 on Bone Are Enhanced by Zinc

The combination of nutritional factors may have additive or synergistic effects in the prevention of bone loss with increasing age. Zinc has been shown to enhance effect of MK-7 in increasing bone calcium content *in vivo* [232]. Rats were orally administered either vehicle (distilled water), zinc sulfate (10 mg Zn/kg body weight), MK-7 (5 mg/kg), or zinc (10 mg/kg) plus MK-7 (5 mg/kg) once a day for 7 days [232]. Femoral dry weight was singificantly increased after the administration of both zinc and MK-7, although a significant change was not seen after the administration of zinc or MK-7 alone. Calcium content in the femoral-diaphyseal and metaphyseal tissues was significantly increased after zinc administration. Such an increase was not found after MK-7 alone. Bone calcium content was synergistically enhanced after the administration of both zinc and MK-7. Alkaline phosphatase activity and DNA content in the diaphyseal and metaphyseal tissues were significantly increased after the administration of zinc or MK-7; these increases were additively enhanced by both zinc and MK-7.

Likewise, the intake of supplement containing both zinc (16.75 mg/kg) and MK-7 (16.88 μg/kg) once a day for 15 days caused additive or synergistic increases in femoral dry weight, alkaline phosphatase activity, DNA, calcium and zinc contents in the diaphyseal and metaphyseal tissues [232].

This study demonstrates that the administration of both zinc and MK-7 can enhance additively or synergistically bone components in female elderly rats, suggesting a role in the prevention of osteoporosis with increasing age. The supplemental intake with combination of MK-7 and zinc may be useful in the prevention and treatment of osteoporosis with increasing age.

Dietary MK-7 Intake Increases Osteocalcin Production in Human Subjects

Epidemiologic data indicate that intake of *natto* may play a role in the prevention of osteoporosis [204]. However, it has been not determined whether prolonged intake of dietary natto causes an increase in MK-7 and a corresponding increase in γ-carboxylated osteocalcin in the serum of normal individuals.

The change in circulating MK-7 and γ-carboxylated osteocalcin (Gla osteocalcin) concentrations in normal individuals with the intake of fermented soybean (*natto*) has been shown [233, 234]. Forty-eight volunteers (45 men and 3 women) were divided into three groups of 16 volunteers each (15 men and 1 women), and each group was given sequentially fermented soybeans (50 g) containing three different amounts of MK-7 once a day for 14 days as follows: either regular natto with MK-7 865 μg/100 g diet of *natto*, reinforced *natto* containing MK-7 1295 μg/100 g, or MK-7 1730 μg/100 g [233]. Serum MK-7 was not found in normal individuals who had not eaten *natto*.

Serum MK-7 and γ-carboxylated osteocalcin concentrations were significantly raised 7, 10, and 14 days after the start of intake of reinforced natto containing MK-7 1295 or 1730 μg/100 g [234]. Serum γ-carboxylated osteocalcin levels were not significantly elevated with intake of regular *natto*, although serum MK-7 levels were significantly raised. Moreover, serum γ-carboxylated osteocalcin concentration was significantly elevated 14 days after the intake of *natto* containing either 1295 or 1730 μg of MK-7/100 g diets as compared with that after regular *natto* intake [234]. The intake of dietary MK-7 in reinforced *natto* can stimulate γ-carboxylation of osteocalcin, which plays an important role in bone formation in normal human subjects.

Appropriate amount of dietary MK-7 may have stimulatory effects on bone mineralization in those individuals. Intake of reinforced *natto* that contains more MK-7 than regular *natto* may participate in prevention of age-related bone loss.

The effect of MK-7 supplementation on osteocalcin carboxylation in healthy prepubertal children has been shown [233, 234]. Objective was to study effect of 45 μg MK-7 on the circulating levels of undercarboxylated osteocalcin (ucOC) and carboxylated osteocalcin (cOC) in healthy prepubertal children. This study was double-blind randomized placebo-controlled trial in determining the effect of MK-7 supplementation on the carboxylation of osteocalcin in healthy children (*n*=55) for 8 weeks. Serum levels of ucOc, oOC, and MK-7 were measured at baseline and after 8 weeks, together with bone markers and coagulation parameters. The ucOc:cOc ratio (UCR) was used as an indicator of vitamin K status. In the MK-7-supplemented group (*n*=28), the circulating concentration of inactive ucOC reduced and UCR improved whereas the concentration of MK-7 increased. Within placebo group, ucOC, cOC, UCR, and MK-7 did not significantly change over time. In both groups, bone markers and coagulation parameters remained constant over time. These findings demonstate that modest supplementation with MK-7 increases circulating concentration of MK-7 and increases osteocalcin carboxylation in healthy and prepubertal children. Thus, dietary intake of MK-7 has been shown to have treatment effects on bone loss in human subjects with increasing age.

Moreover, despite contradictory data on vitamin K supplementation and bone health, the European Food Safety Authorities (EFSA) accepted the health claim on vitamin K's role in maintenance of normal bone. In line with EFSA's opinion, supplementation with 3-year high-dose vitamin K_1 (phylloquinone) and K_2 (short-chain menaquinone-4) has been shown to improve bone health after menopause [235]. Because of the longer half-life and greater potency of the long-chain MK-7, Knapen *et al.* have extended these investigations by measuring the effect of low-dose MK-7 supplementation on bone health. Healthy postmenopausal women (n = 244) received for 3 years placebo or MK-7 (180 μg MK-7/day) capsules [235]. Bone mineral density of lumbar spine, total hip, and femoral neck was measured by DXA; bone strength indices of the femoral neck were calculated. Vertebral fracture assessment was performed by DXA and used as measure for vertebral fractures. Circulating uncarboxylated osteocalcin (ucOC) and carboxylated OC (cOC) were measured; the ucOC/cOC ratio served as marker of vitamin K status [235]. Measurements occurred at baseline and after 1, 2, and 3 years of treatment. MK-7 intake significantly improved vitamin K status and decreased the age-related decline in BMC and BMD at the lumbar spine and femoral neck, but not at the total hip [235]. Bone strength was also favorably affected by MK-7. MK-7 significantly decreased the loss in vertebral height of the lower thoracic region at the mid-site of the vertebrae [235]. MK-7 supplements may help postmenopausal women to prevent bone loss. Whether these results can be extrapolated to other populations, e.g., children and men, needs further investigation [235].

Conclusion

Vitamin K_2, which is co-factor of γ-carboxylase that glutamate residues of osteocalcin are converted into γ-carboxyglutamate, has been shown to stimulate production of osteocalcin. Vitamin K_2 has been shown to inhibit osteoclastic bone resorption and stimulate osteoblastic bone formation, thereby increasing bone mass and preventing bone loss. Intake of dietary vitamin K_2 has been shown to stimulate γ-carboxylation of osteocalcin in normal human subjects and increase bone mineral density and prevent bone fracture. Dietary vitamin K_2 may be useful in the treatment of osteoporosis.

The molecular mechanism by which vitamin K_2 stimulates bone mass may be partly mediated through the pathways of Ca^{2+}- and cyclic AMP-dependent signalings in osteoclast and the downregulating basal and cytokine-induced NF-κB activation, by increasing IκB mRNA, in a γ-carboxylation-independent manner. Vitamin K_2 may regulate a transcription of bone-specific genes that act through steroid and xenobiotic receptors (SXRs) to promote expression of osteoblastic markers, and it stimulates protein synthesis including osteocalcin in osteoblastic cells. Further studies remain to be elucidated. Vitamin K_2, which was discovered as blood coagulation factor, may have multifunctional roles in the living body.

Chapter 6

Satuma Mandarin Orange β-Cryptoxanthin and Osteoporosis Treatment

Vitamin A (retinol, retinal and retinoic acid) has been shown to have a role in the regulation of bone cells and it may have an anabolic effect on bone [236-238]. However, vitamin A is also known to have a detrimental effect on bone at high doses [239-242]. In laboratory animals, high levels of vitamin A lead to accelerated bone resorption, bone fractures, and osteoporotic bone lesions [239].

There is growing evidence that carotenoids, which are a provitamin A, have an anabolic effect on bone metabolism. Carotenoids (carotene and xanthophyll) are present in fruit and vegetables. β-Cryptoxanthin, a kind of xanthophyll, is abundant in Satsuma mandarin orange (*Citrus unshiu* MARC.). Of various carotenoids, β-cryptoxanthin has been found to have a unique anabolic effect on bone due to stimulating osteoblastic bone formation and inhibiting osteoclastic bone resorption [243, 244].

This chapter has been written to outline the recent advances concerning the role of vitamin A, lycopene andβ-cryptoxanthin in the regulation of bone homeostasis and in the prevention of osteoporosis. The cellular and molecular mechanisms by which β-cryptoxanthin stimulates osteoblastic bone formation and inhibits osteoclastic bone resorption are reviewed, especially.

Carotenoids and Bone Homeostasis

Carotene is generically named for carotene (α, β, γ, δ, ε) and lycopene, which are a natural compound with the derivative of fundamental form of $C_{40}H_{56}$ in chemical structure. Carotene is contained in plant and fruits. Other derivatives with hydroxyl group for $C_{40}H_{56}$ are named as xanthophyll, which are lutein, zeaxanthin, canthaxanthin, fucoxanthin, antheraxanthin, violaxanthin and β-cryptoxanthin. Carotenoids are named generically for carotene and xanthophyll.

The effects of carotenes, canthaxanthin, fucoxanthin, antheraxanthin and violaxanthin on bone homeostasis have not been clearly shown. Among various carotenes and xanthophylls (includingβ-carotene, lycopene, lutein, astaxanthin andβ-cryptoxanthin), β-cryptoxanthin has been found to have a unique anabolic effect on bone calcification *in vitro* [243, 244].

Myricetin, kaempferol, isorhamnetin, curcumin, hesperidin or rutin (quercetin-3-rutinoside) of various flavonoids does not have an effect on bone formation and calcification *in vitro* [244].

Lycopene and Bone Homeostasis

The chemical structure of lycopene is shown in Figure 13. Lycopene has been shown to have an inhibitory effect on bone resorption *in vitro* [245], although lycopene has not been shown to have a stimulatory effect on mineralization using rat femoral tissues *in vitro* [243]. Osteoclasts produce reactive oxygen species (ROS) that can stimulate bone resorption. Lycopene (10^{-5} M) has been found to inhibit basal and parathyroid hormone (PTH)-stimulated osteoclastic mineral resorption and formation of tartrate-resistant acid phosphatase (TRAP) activity-possitive multinucleated osteoclasts, as well as the ROS produced by osteoclastic cells prepared from bone marrow of rat femur [245]. Lycopene may have an inhibitory effect on osteoclastic bone resorption, suggesting that lycopene has a role in the prevention of osteoporosis.

In a cross-sectional study by using 33 postmenopausal women aged 50-60 years, groups with higher lycopene intake, as determined from the dietary records, showed higher serum lycopene [246]. A higher serum lycopene has been found to be associated with a low cross-linked *N*-telopeptides of type I collagen [246]. Similarly, groups with higher serum lycopene have lower protein oxidation [246]. These observations suggest that the dietary antioxidant lycopene reduces oxidative stress and the levels of bone turnover markers in postmenopausal women, and may be beneficial in reducing the risk of osteoporosis [246].

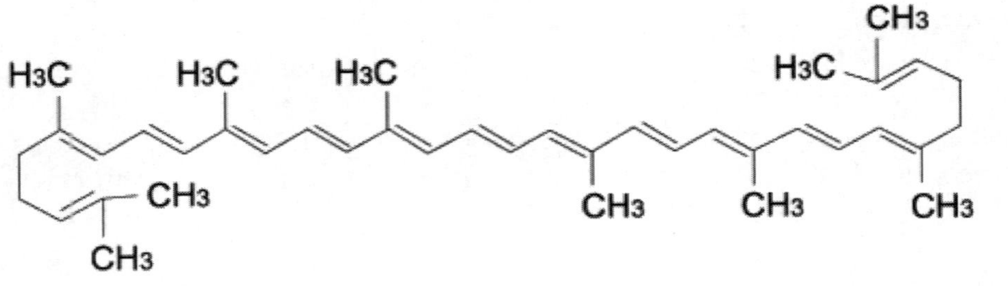

Figure 13. Chemical structure of lycopene. The molecular weight of lycopene ($C_{40}H_{56}$) is 536.87.

Postmenopausal women supplemented with lycopene have been shown to increase antioxidant capacity and decrease oxidative stress and the bone resorption marker *N*-telopeptide [247]. Lycopene decreases bone resorption markers and may reduce the risk of osteoporosis [247]. Sixty postmenopausal women, 50-60 years old, were recruited [247]. Following a 1-month washout without lycopene consumption, participants consumed either regular tomato juice, lycopene-rich tomato juice, tomato lycopene capsules, or placebo capsules, twice daily for total lycopene intakes of 30, 70, 30, and 0 mg/day respectively for 4 months [247]. Lycopene supplementation for 4 months significantly increased serum lycopene and decreased lipid peroxidation, and cross-linked aminoterminal *N*-telopeptide as compared to placebo [247]. These findings suggest that the antioxidant lycopene is beneficial in reducing oxidative stress parameters and the bone resorption marker [247].

The intake of dietary lycopene may have a role in the prevention of osteoporosis.

Vitamin A and Bone Homeostasis

Vitamin A (retinol, retinal and retinoic acid) is formed from carotenoids, which are provitamin A, in the animals and humans. The chemical structure of vitamin A is shown in Figure 14. The retinoic acid receptors α, β and γ (RARα, RARβ and RARγ) are nuclear hormone receptors that regulate fundamental processes during embryogenesis, but their roles in skeletal development and growth are investigated.

Mice deficients in RARα and RARγ (or RARβ and RARγ) have been shown to exhibit severe growth retardation obvious by about 3 weeks postnatally [236]. Their growth plates were defective and, importantly, display a major drop in aggrecan expression and content [236]. Mice deficients in RARα and RARβ, however, were virtually normal, suggesting that RARγ is essential [236]. RARγ is the most strongly expressed RAR in mouse growth plate and its expression characterizes the proliferative and pre-hypertrophic zones where aggrecan is strongly expressed also [236]. Retinoic acid receptors may be required for skeletal growth, matrix homeostasis and growth plate function in postnatal mouse, suggesting a role of retinoic acid in bone growth [236].

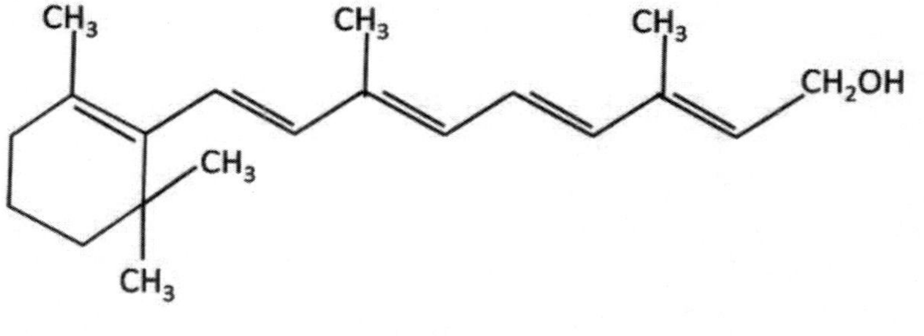

Figure 14. Chemical structure of vitamin A. The molecular weight of vitamin A ($C_{20}H_{30}O$) is 286.46.

The action of retinol and carotene on bone cells is shown *in vitro* by evaluating cell growth, alkaline phosphatase activity and the mRNA expression of a differentiation marker protein of osteoblastic cells [237]. The clonal osteogenic cell line MC3T3-E1, which was established from newborn mouse calvaria, has a capacity of differentiation into osteoblast and mineralization *in vitro* [237]. Retinol and β-carotene have been shown to inhibit the proliferation of MC3T3-E1 cells as well as DNA synthesis of the cells in a dose-dependent manner [237]. Retinol and β-carotene induced differentiation of the MC3T3-E1 cells by increasing alkaline phosphatase activity dose dependently [237]. Osteopontin is one of the matrix proteins in osteoblasts. Retinol and β-carotene caused an increase in the expression of osteopontin mRNA [237]. α-Carotene, canthaxanthin and lycopene also have been shown to inhibit MC3T3-E1 cell proliferation and to increase alkaline phosphatase activity and osteopontin mRNA expression [237]. Retinol and carotenoids may have a direct stimulatory effect on the differentiation of osteoblasts at the physiological concentration [237].

The effects of retinoids on osteoclast differentiation in cultured mouse bone marrow cells (BMCs), bone marrow macrophages (BMMs), spleen cells, and RAW264.7 cells have been examined by analyzing osteoclast formation and expression of genes important in signal transduction and osteoclast function [238]. All-*trans*-retinoic acid (ATRA) did not stimulate osteoclastogenesis in BMCs, but inhibited hormone and RANKL-induced gene expression and formation of osteoclasts [238]. In BMMs, spleen cells, and RAW264.7 cells, osteoclast differentiation and formation stimulated by M-CSF/RANKL were inhibited by ATRA [238]. ATRA also abolished an increase in the transcription factors c-Fos and NFAT2 stimulated by RANKL and suppressed down-regulation of the anti-osteoclastogenic transcription factor MafB [238]. These findings suggest that the activation of RAR by retinoids in myeloid hematopoietic precursor cells decreases osteoclast formation by altering expression of the transcription factors c-Fos, NFAT2, and MafB [238].

The excessive intakes of vitamin A have been shown to have adverse skeletal effects in animals [248]. High vitamin A intake may lead to an increased risk of fracture in humans. A total of 75.747 women from the Women's Health Initiative Observational Study were participated in this study. The risk of hip and total fractures was determined using Cox proportional hazards models according to different intakes of vitamin A and retinol [248]. In the analysis adjusted for some covariates (age; protein, vitamin D, vitamin K, calcium, caffeine, and alcohol intakes; body mass index; hormone therapy use; smoking; metabolic equivalents hours per week; ethnicity; and region of clinical center), the association between vitamin A intake and the risk of fracture was not statistically significant [248]. Analyses for retinol showed similar trends. When the interaction term was analyzed as categorical, the highest intake of retinol with vitamin D was significant [248]. Women with lower vitamin D intake (< 11 microgram/day) in the highest quintile of intake of both vitamin A and retinol had a modest increased risk of total fracture [248]. No association between vitamin A or retinol intake and the risk of hip or total fractures was observed in postmenopausal women [248]. Only a modest increase in total fracture risk with high vitamin A and retinol intakes may be observed in the low vitamin D-intake group [248].

Association between vitamin D deficiency and excess of vitamin A as a potential risk factor of osteoporosis and fracture has been shown [237]. Whereas in women with vitamin D deficiency the risk of osteoporosis increased was up 5 times higher than women in the lowest quintile of retinol [237]. High retinol levels together with vitamin D deficiency may be hitherto an overlooked risk factor for osteoporosis.

Previous epidemiological studies that are conducted in retinol-supplemented subjects show an association between high serum levels or dietary intake of retinol and risk of hip fracture [239]. On the other side, observational studies revealed that non-supplemented subjects with higher dietary intake of retinol loosed less bone with age than subjects with lower intake. This discrepancy suggests that nutrition plays a major role in conditioning the effects of retinol on bone [239].

Retinol is derived from both retinoids, which are contained in animal food, and carotenoids, which are contained in vegetables and fruits. A possible role of carotenoids in involutional osteoporosis was evaluated. When plasma levels of β-carotene and other carotenoids, in addition to those of retinol, were measured in free-living, non-supplemented, elderly women with or without severe osteoporosis, plasma levels of retinol and of all carotenoids tested, with the exception of lutein, were consistently lower in osteoporotic than in control women [239]. A weak association was found only between retinol and femoral neck bone mineral density in osteoporotic women [239]. A bone sparing effect of retinol, to which the provitamin A activity of some carotenoids, may be contributed [239].

β-Cryptoxanthin and Bone Homeostasis

Xanthophyllβ-cryptoxanthin, which is a kind of carotenoid, is abundant in Satsuma mandarin orange (*Citrus unshiu* MARC). The chemical structure of β-cryptoxanthin is shown in Figure 15. The biological function ofβ-cryptoxanthin in animal and human, however, has been not determined fully. The author found that β-cryptoxanthin has been shown to have a unique anabolic effect on bone calcification; such an effect is not seen in lutein, lycopene, or astaxanthin, which is other carotenoids and flavonoid rutin (quercetin-3-rutinoside) [243, 244].

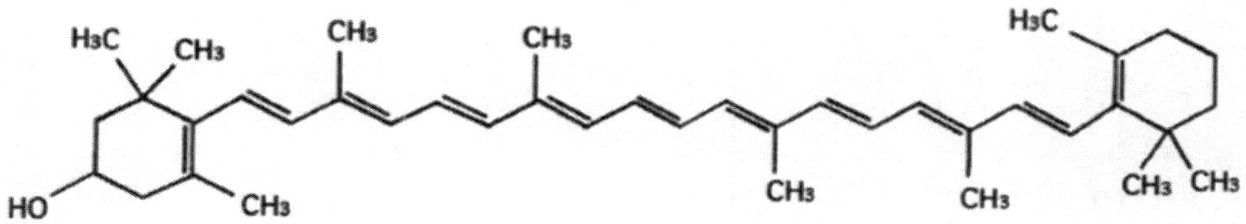

Figure 15. Chemical structure of β -cryptoxanthin. The molecular weight of this compound ($C_{40}H_{56}O$) is 552. β -Cryptoxanthin is a kind of carotenoid that is abundant in Satsuma mandarin (*Citrus unshiu* MARC.).

β-Cryptoxanthin Stimulates Bone Formation and Inhibits Bone Resorption in Tissue Culture

β-Cryptoxanthin has been shown to have a unique anabolic effect on bone calcification. Culture with β-cryptoxanthin (10^{-7} or 10^{-6} M) has been found to induce a significant increase in calcium content and alkaline phosphatase activity in the femoral-diaphyseal (cortical bone) and -metaphyseal (trabecular bone) tissues *in vitro*. Lutein, lycopene, and rutin (10^{-8} to 10^{-6} M) did not have anabolic effects on alkaline phosphatase activity and calcium contents in rat femoral-diaphyseal and -metaphyseal tissues [243]. Astaxanthin and β-carotene (10^{-6} or 10^{-5} M) did not have an effect on the femoral calcium contents [244]. Myricetin, kaempferol, isorhamnetin, curcumin or hesperidin (10^{-7} to 10^{-5} M) had no effect on bone calcium content in tissue cultures *in vitro* [244]. Quercetin significantly increased calcium content in the femoral diaphyseal tissues but not metaphyseal tissues. Alkaline phosphatase is known to participate in mineralization in the bone tissues.β-Cryptoxanthin has a unique anabolic effect on bone calcification *in vitro*. The effect of β-cryptoxanthin increasing bone components was completely prevented in the presence of cycloheximide, an inhibitor of protein synthesis, suggesting that the effect is needed newly protein synthesis [244].

β-Cryptoxanthin has also been shown to inhibit bone resorption in femoral bone tissue cultures *in vitro* [244]. Parathyroid hormone (PTH) or prostaglandin E_2 (PGE_2), which is a bone-resorbing factor, can stimulate osteoclastic bone resorption *in vitro* [162-164]. Culture with PTH or PGE_2 caused a significant decrease in calcium content in the diaphyseal and metaphyseal tissues [244]. This decrease was completely inhibited in the presence of β-cryptoxanthin (10^{-8} to 10^{-6} M). Likewise, culture with β-cryptoxanthin completely inhibited PTH- or PGE_2-induced increase in medium glucose consumption and lactic acid production by bone tissues [244]. β-Cryptoxanthin has an inhibitory effect on bone resorption in bone tissue culture *in vitro*.

Thus, β-cryptoxanthin has been shown to have stimulatory effects on osteoblastic bone formation and inhibitory effects on osteoclastic bone resorption in bone tissue culture *in vitro*.

It has been reported that the serum concentration of β-cryptoxanthin due to consumption of vegetable juice in women is in the range of 1.3×10^{-7} to 5.3×10^{-7} M [249]. β-Cryptoxanthin in the range of 10^{-8} to 10^{-6} M had a significant anabolic effect on biochemical components in rat femoral tissues *in vitro*, suggesting a physiologic role in the regulation of bone metabolism.

β-Cryptoxanthin Stimulates Gene Expression in Osteoblastic Cells

The cellular and molecular mechanisms by whichβ-cryptoxanthin stimulates bone formation in bone tissues have been examined using osteoblastic MC3T3-E1 cells *in vitro*. β-Cryptoxanthin has been found to stimulate the proliferation of osteoblastic cells in subconfluent monolayers in a medium containing 10% fetal bovine serum [250]. Culture with β-cryptoxanthin also caused a significant increase in biochemical components (alkaline phosphatase activity, protein and DNA contents) of osteoblastic cells [250]. This effect was significantly abolished in the presence of staurosporine, an inhibitor of protein kinase C, or PD98059, an inhibitor of mitosis activated protein kinase (MAP) kinase, although the effect ofβ-cryptoxanthin in increasing cellular biochemical components was not significantly prevented after culture with dibucain, an inhibitor of Ca^{2+}/calmodulin-dependent protein kinase [250]. The stimulatory effects of β-cryptoxanthin on osteoblastic cell components seem to be partly mediated through signaling factors of protein kinase C or MAP kinase in the cells.

The effects of β-cryptoxanthin in increasing the biochemical components in osteoblastic cells were completely inhibited in the presence of 5,6-dichloro-1-β-D-ribofuranosylbenzimidazole (DRB), an inhibitor of RNA polymerase II, suggesting that the effect of carotenoid results from a stimulatory effect on transcriptional activity in osteoblastic cells.

The mineralization in osteoblastic cells has been shown to stimulate after prolonged culture with β-cryptoxanthin [251]. The stimulatory effects ofβ-cryptoxanthin on mineralization may result from the carotenoid-induced proliferation and differentiation of osteoblastic cells.

β-Cryptoxanthin may stimulate gene expression for proteins that are involved in bone formation and mineralization in osteoblastic cells. The effect of β-cryptoxanthin on gene expression in osteoblastic cells using reverse transcription-polymerase chain reaction (RT-PCR) has been examined. Culture with β-cryptoxanthin was found to stimulate the mRNA expression of IGF-I or TGF-β1 in osteoblastic cells [250]. This finding may support the view thatβ-cryptoxanthin has a stimulatory effect on transcriptional activity in osteoblastic cells. IGF-I or TGF-β1 is a bone growth factor produced from osteoblasts [252, 253]. The stimulatory effect of β-cryptoxanthin on the proliferation of osteoblastic cells may be partly mediated through the action of IGF-I or TGF-β1 produced from the cells.

β-Cryptoxanthin (10^{-7} or 10^{-6} M) has been found to increase the mRNA expression of Runx2, α1 (I) collagen, and alkaline phosphatase in osteoblastic MC3T3-E1 cells [251]. Runx2 (Cbfa1) is a member of the runt domain family of transcription factors and a master regulator of osteoblast differentiation [254]. α1 (I) Collagen is a matrix protein that is related to bone formation and mineralization in osteoblast lineage cells [159]. Alkaline phosphatase participates in the mineralization process in osteoblastic cells [255].β-Cryptoxanthin had a stimulatory effect on the gene expression of for various proteins involved in osteoblasic bone formation [251].

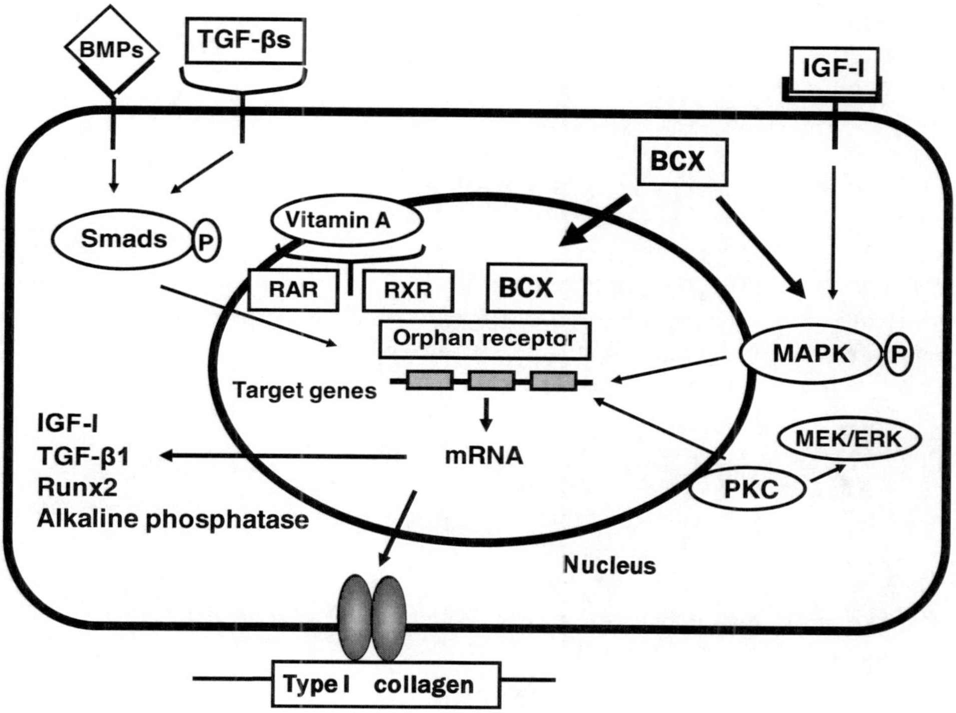

Figure 16. Cellular and molecular mechanisms by which β -cryptoxanthin (BCX) stimulates bone formation and mineralization in osteoblastic cells. BCX may bind to orphan receptors in the nucleus of osteoblastic cells, and it stimulates gene expression of bone formation-related proteins. BCX also stimulates nuclear transcriptional activity mediated through activation of protein kinase C (PKC) or mitosis activated protein kinase (MAPK) in osteoblastic cells.

The effects of β-cryptoxanthin in stimulating Runx2, α1 (I) collagen, and alkaline phosphatase mRNA expression in osteoblastic MC3T3-E1 cells has been shown to prevent in the presence of DRB [251], supporting the view that the carotenoid stimulates transcriptional activity in osteoblastic MC3T3-E1 cells.

Vitamin A (retinol) may be able to bind to nuclear receptors in cells. Retinol andβ-carotene has been shown to inhibit the proliferation of osteoblastic MC3T3-E1 cells as well as DNA synthesis of the cells, due to increasing alkaline phosphatase activity dose dependently (10^{-9} to 10^{-7} M) [237]. Vitamin A (10^{-7} or 10^{-6} M) increased alkaline phosphatase activity in osteoblastic cells [251]. β-Cryptoxanthin (10^{-7} or 10^{-6} M) caused a significant increase in alkaline phosphatase activity and protein content in osteoblastic cells. This effect was also seen in the presence of vitamin A (10^{-6} M) [251]. Moreover, the stimulatory effects of β-cryptoxanthin on the expression of Runx2 type 1 and α1 (I) collagen mRNA were observed in the presence of vitamin A [251]. Vitamin A did not have a significant effect on Runx2 type 1 mRNA expression in osteoblastic MC3T3-E1 cells [251]. Thus, the mode of action of β-cryptoxanthin on gene expression in osteoblastic cells may differ from that of vitamin A, which is mediated through the RXR receptor in the nucleus of the cells [251].

It has been speculated that β-cryptoxanthin may be able to bind other receptors (including orphan receptors that ligands are not unknown), and that the carotenoid may stimulate transcriptional activity in osteoblastic cells. The mechanism by whichβ-cryptoxanthin stimulates proliferation, differentiation, and mineralization in osteoblastic cells is summarized in Figure 16.

β-Cryptoxanthin Suppresses Osteoclastogenesis and Osteoclastic Cell Function

β-Cryptoxanthin Inhibits Osteoclastogenesis

The receptor activator of nuclear factor-kappa B (NF-κB) ligand (RANKL) plays a pivotal role in osteoclastogenesis from bone marrow cells. RANKL expression is induced in osteoblastic cells and bone marrow stromal cells in response to osteoporotic factors, such as PTH, PGE_2, and 1, 25-dihydroxyvitamin D_3 [1, 25$(OH)_2D_3$], and combined treatment of hematopoietic cells with macrophage colony-stimulating factor (M-CSF), and the soluble form of RANKL (sRANKL) induce osteoclast differentiation *in vitro* [77, 78]. The receptor protein RANK (receptor activator of NF-κB) is expressed on the surface of osteoclast progenitors.

β-Cryptoxanthin (10^{-8} to 10^{-6} M) has been shown to have a potent inhibitory effect on osteoclast-like cell formation in mouse marrow culture *in vitro* [256]. The inhibitory effect of β-cryptoxanthin on osteoclast-like cell formation was seen at the later stage of osteoclast differentiation in bone marrow cultures [256]. Culture with β-cryptoxanthin caused a marked inhibition of osteoblast-like cell formation induced in the presence of PTH, PGE_2, 1, 25$(OH)_2D_3$, lipopolysaccharide or tumor necrosis factor-α (TNF-α). β-Cryptoxanthin also had a significant inhibitory effect on osteoclast-like cell formation induced by RANKL [256]. The inhibitory effect of β-cryptoxanthin was equal to that of 17β-estradiol (E_2), calcitonin, genistein and zinc sulfate, which can inhibit osteoclast-like cell formation induced by bone-resorbing factors [256].

The interaction of RANKL with its receptor RANK leads to the recruitment of the signaling adaptor molecules TRAFs (TNF receptor-associated factors) to the receptor complex and the activation of NF-κB and c-Jun N-terminal kinase (JNK) [257, 258]. Protein kinase C family enzyme has a role in the regulation of osteoclast formation and function potentially by participating in the extracellular signaling-regulated kinase (ERK) signaling pathway of M-CSF and RANKL [258].

Phorbol 12-myristate 13-acetate (PMA), an activator of protein kinase C, stimulated osteoclast-like cell formation in mouse marrow cultures, and PMA-induced osteoclastogenesis was found to inhibit in the presence of β-cryptoxanthin [156]. Moreover, β-cryptoxanthin had a significant inhibitory effect on dibutyryl cyclic adenosine monophosphate (DcAMP)-induced osteoclast-like cell formation in mouse marrow cultures [256]. It is assumed that activation of protein kinase C and protein kinase A pathways leads to increased RANKL expression, and thatβ-cryptoxanthin can inhibit protein kinase C- or protein kinase A-related RANKL expression in osteoclastogenesis.

β-Cryptoxanthin Stimulates Apoptosis and Suppresses Osteoclastic Cell Function

The effects of β-cryptoxanthin on mature osteoclasts have been examined [259]. M-CSF-dependent bone marrow macrophages were cultured in the presence of M-CSF and RANKL for 4 days [259]. The osteoclastic cells formed were further cultured in medium containing β-cryptoxanthin with or without M-CSF and RANKL for 24-72 hours. The number of osteoclastic cells has been found to decrease after culture with β-cryptoxanthin (10^{-7} or 10^{-6} M) in the presence or absence of M-CSF and RANKL for 72 hours. β-Cryptoxanthin-induced decrease in osteoclastic cells was significantly inhibited in the presence of caspase-3 inhibitor. The results of agarose gel electrophoresis showed the presence of low-molecular-weight DNA fragments of adherent cells cultured with β-cryptoxanthin. These findings indicate that the carotenoid induces apoptotic cell death.

Apoptosis-related gene expression was determined using RT-PCR [259]. The expression of caspase-3 mRNA or Apaf-2, which involves apoptosis, in osteoclastic cells was found to stimulate after culture with β-cryptoxanthin in the prsence or absence of M-CSF and RANKL [259]. β-Cryptoxanthin-induced apoptotic cell death may be partly mediated through caspase-3 expression in osteoclastic cells.

The expression of Bcl-2 mRNA, which is involved in rescue of apoptosis, was significantly decreased after culture withβ-cryptoxanthin in the presence or absence of M-CSF and RANKL [259]. However, Akt-1 mRNA expression was not significantly changed in culture with β-cryptoxanthin. The decrease in Bcl-2 mRNA expression may partly contribute to the effect of β-cryptoxanthin in stimulating the apoptotic cell death of osteoclastic cells.

Culture with β-cryptoxanthin has been found to have suppressive effects on tartrate-resistant acid phosphatase (TRACP) activity, and it decreases TRACP and cathepsin K mRNA expressions in osteoclastic cells in the presence or absence of M-CSF and RANKL [259]. These findings suggest thatβ-cryptoxanthin inhibits the enhancement of bone-resorbing activity in osteoclasts. β-Cryptoxanthin inhibitd various bone-resorbing factors-induced decrease in bone calcium content and increase in lactic acid production in rat femoral tisuue culture system *in vitro*. Presumably, β-cryptoxanthin has an inhibitory effect on the activation of mature osteoclasts.

β-Cryptoxanthin has been demonstrated to have stimulatory effects on apoptotic cell death due to activating gene expression of its related proteins. The carotenoid also has suppressive effects on TRACP activity and gene expression of enzymes that involve in bone-resorbing activity in osteoclastic cells. The action of β-cryptoxanthin in osteoclasts is summarized in Figure 17.

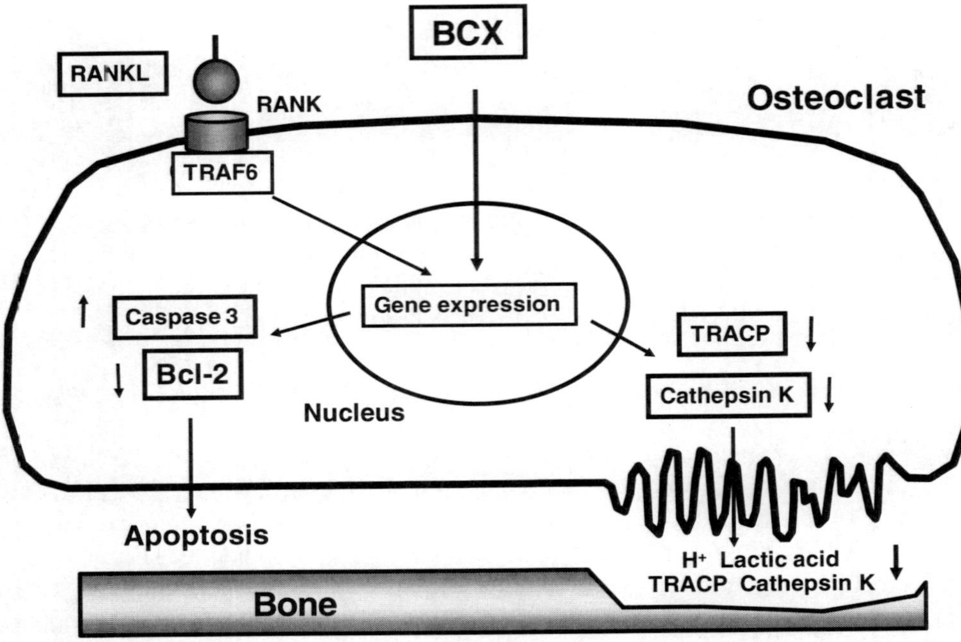

Figure 17. The molecular mechanism by which β -cryptoxanthin (BCX) has suppressive effects on mature osteoclasts. BCX stimulates apoptotic cell death by stimulating the gene expression of caspase-3, a apotosis-inducing enzyme, and suppression of gene expression of Bcl-2, a rescue protein of apoptosis. Additionally, BCX suppresses gene expression of TRACP and cathepsin K, which are bone resorption-related enzymes, and their enzyme activities in mature osteoclasts.

Anabolic Effect of β-Cryptoxanthin on Bone Is Synergistically Enhanced by Zinc

Zinc, an essential trace element, has been shown to have anabolic effects due to stimulating osteoblastic bone formation and osteoclastic bone resorption *in vitro* and *in vivo* [141-144]. Zinc has been shown to enhance the anabolic effects of β-cryptoxanthin on bone.

Combination of β-Cryptoxanthin and Zinc Has a Synergistic Effect in Bone Tissues in Vitro

The effect of the combination of β-cryptoxanthin and zinc sulfate on bone components in the femoral-diaphyseal and -metaphyseal tissues of young rats *in vitro* has been examined [260]. Bone tissues were cultured for 48 hours in a serum-free medium containing either vegicle, β-cryptoxanthin (10^{-9} - 10^{-7} M) or zinc sulfate (10^{-6} - 10^{-4} M). The presence of β-cryptoxanthin (10^{-9} M) or zinc (10^{-6} M) did not have a significant effect on calcium content in the femoral-diaphyseal or -metaphyseal tissue [260]. However, culture with combination of β-cryptoxanthin (10^{-9} M) and zinc (10^{-6} M) caused a significant increase in calcium content in the femoral-diaphyseal and -metaphyseal tissues. Such an effect was not observed with the combination of β-cryptoxanthin (10^{-9} M) plus genistein (10^{-6} M) or menaquinone-7 (10^{-6} M), or zinc (10^{-6} M) plus genistein (10^{-6} M) or menaquinone-7 (10^{-6} M) [260].

The combination of β-cryptoxanthin (10^{-9} M) plus zinc (10^{-6} M) caused a remarkable increase in alkaline phosphatase activity and DNA content in the diaphyseal and metaphyseal tissues, while their application alone did not have an effect on the enzyme activity or DNA content in the bone tissues [260]. The effect of the combination of β-cryptoxanthin (10^{-9} M) plus zinc (10^{-6} M) in increasing alkaline phosphatase activity, DNA and calcium contents in the diaphyseal and metaphyseal tissues was completely prevented in the presence of cycloheximide (10^{-6} M), an inhibitor of protein synthesis, or DBR, an inhibitor of transcriptional activity [260].

Effect of β-Cryptoxanthin in Osteoblastic Cells Is Enhanced by Zinc

The effect of the combination withβ-cryptoxanthin and zinc or other factors [including 1, 25-dihydroxyvitamin D_3 [1, 25$(OH)_2D_3$], 17β-estradiol, genistein, or menaquinone-7 (MK-7)] on gene expression in osteoblastic MC3T3-E1 cells has been examined [261]. Culture withβ-cryptoxanthin (10^{-7} or 10^{-6} M) caused a significant increase in the expression of Runx2 and alkaline phosphatase mRNAs in the cells. This effect was not enhanced in the presence of 1, 25$(OH)_2D_3$, 17β-estradiol, genistein, or MK-7. Culture with zinc sulfate (10^{-5} M) caused a significant increase in α 1(I) collagen mRNA expression, while it did not have a significant effect on Runx2 or osteocalcin mRNA expression in the cells. The effect ofβ-cryptoxanthin (10^{-7} M) in increasing Runx2 or α1(I) collagen mRNA expressions was significantly enhanced in the presence of zinc (10^{-6} or 10^{-5} M) [261]. This effect was not seen in the presence of cycloheximide or DRB. The additive and/or synergistic effect ofβ-cryptoxanthin and zinc on gene expression in osteoblastic cells is partly resulted in newly synthesized protein components.

Zinc has been shown to activate aminoacyl-tRNA synthetase, a rate-limiting enzyme, in the translational process of protein synthesis [53-56]. β-Cryptoxanthin can stimulate transcriptional activity in osteoblastic cells [250, 251]. It has been speculated thatβ-cryptoxanthin stimulates gene expression and zinc increases translational activity in osteoblastic cells. This may be important as a possible mechanism by which zinc enhances the anabolic effect ofβ-cryptoxanthin in osteoblastic cells.

Effect of β-Cryptoxanthin in Osteoclastic Cells Is Synergistically Enhanced by Zinc

The effect ofβ-cryptoxanthin on osteoclastic cells formed in the mouse marrow culture system *in vitro* has been found to enhance after culture with zinc [262]. Bone marrow cells were isolated from mice. The macrophage colony-stimulating factor (M-CSF)-dependent bone marrow cells were cultured in the presence of M-CSF (10 ng/ml) and receptor activator of nuclear factor-κB (NF-κB) ligand (RANKL; 50 ng/ml) for 96 hours. The osteoclastic cells formed were further cultured for 24 or 72 hours in a medium containing either vehicle, β-cryptoxanthin, zinc sulfate, orβ-cryptoxanthin plus zinc with or without M-CSF (10 ng/ml) and RANKL (50 ng/ml). The number of osteoclastic cells was significantly decreased after culture with the combination ofβ-cryptoxanthin (10^{-7} M) and zinc (10^{-5} M) in the presence or absence of M-CSF and RANKL for 24 or 72 hours as compared with the value forβ-cryptoxanthin or zinc [262].

The results of agarose gel electrophoresis showed the presence of low-molecular weight deoxyribonucleic acid (DNA) fragments of adherent cells cultured withβ-cryptoxanthin (10^{-7} M) plus zinc (10^{-5} M) for 24 or 72 hours in the presence of M-CSF and RANKL, indicating that the combination of the two chemicals synergistically induces apoptotic cell death [54].

β-Cryptoxanthin plus zinc-induced decrease in osteoclastic cells was significantly inhibited in the presence of caspase-3 inhibitor [262]. Culture with β-cryptoxanthin plus zinc for 24 or 72 hours caused a significant increase in caspase-3 mRNA expression in the presence or absence of M-CSF and RANKL as compared with the value for each chemical alone. β-Cryptoxanthin plus zinc-induced increase in caspase-3 mRNA expression was completely inhibited in the presence of cycloheximide or DRB [262]. This suggests that β-cryptoxanthin plus zinc-induced apoptotic cell death is mediated through caspase-3 in osteoclastic cells, and thatβ-cryptoxanthin plus zinc-enhanced caspase-3 mRNA expression in osteoclastic cells is related to newly synthesized protein synthesis.

The mRNA expression of tartrate-resistant acid phosphatase (TRACP) and cathepsin K was significantly decreased after culture with β-cryptoxanthin plus zinc in the presence or absence of M-CSF and RANKL for 72 hours as compared with β-cryptoxanthin or zinc alone [262]. Nuclear factor of activated T cells c1 (NFATc1) mRNA expression was decreased after culture with β-cryptoxanthin plus zinc in the presence or absence of M-CSF and RANKL for 72 hours as compared with each chemical alone, while NF-κB mRNA expression was not changed [262]. TRACP and cathepsin K are enzymes that are involved in the degradation of bone matrix components, and their enzyme activities are increased in RANKL-stimulated bone resorption [77, 78]. It is assumed that the combination ofβ-cryptoxanthin and zinc has a potent-suppressive effect on bone resorption.

NF-κB and NFATc1 are molecules related to RANKL signaling [77, 78]. NFATc1 is a transcriptional factor that enhances the gene expression of TRACP and cathepsin K in osteoclasts, and the binding of NFATc1 to promoter is involved in NF-κkB or AP-1 [77]. It has been speculated that the suppression of NFATc1 mRNA expression induced with the combination ofβ-cryptoxanthin and zinc induces the decrease in NF-κB protein level. This may partly contribute to the decrease in the TRACP or cathepsin K mRNA expression caused by their combination.

The suppressive effects ofβ-cryptoxanthin on osteoclastogenesis have been demonstrated to synergistically enhance in the presence of zinc, and also the combination of β-cryptoxanthin and zinc has potent suppressive effects on osteoclastic cell function *in vitro*.

Anabolic Effect of β-Cryptoxanthin on Bone Is Enhanced by Zinc *In Vivo*

The effects of the combination of β-cryptoxanthin and zinc on bone components in the femoral-diaphyseal (cortical bone) and -metaphyseal (trabecular bone) tissues of rats *in vivo* have been examined [55]. Rats were orally administered either vehicle, β-cryptoxanthin (50 or 100 μg/kg body weight), zinc sulfate (1 or 5 mg Zn/kg), or their combination once a day for 7 days. Alkaline phosphatase activity, DNA and calcium contents in the femaral-diaphyseal tissues were not significantly altered after the administration ofβ-cryptoxanthin

(50 μg/kg) or zinc (1 or 5 mg/kg) [263]. Combined administration ofβ-cryptoxanthin (50 μg/kg) and zinc (1 or 5 mg/kg) caused a synergistic increase in alkaline phosphatase activity, DNA and calcium contents in the diaphyseal tissues [263]. The effect ofβ-cryptoxanthin (50 or 100 μg/kg) in increasing DNA and calcium contents in the metaphyseal tissues was significantly enhanced after the combined administration of zinc (1 or 5 mg/kg), but it did not have a significant effect on the metaphyseal components. The metaphyseal alkaline phosphatase activity has been found to increase markedly after the administration with the combination ofβ-cryptoxanthin (50 μg/kg) and zinc (1 or 5 mg/kg) [263]. This study demonstrates that oral administration with the combination of zinc at lower doses synergistically enhancesβ-cryptoxanthin-induced anabolic effects on bone components in the femoral tissues of rats *in vivo*.

It has been speculated that the combination ofβ-cryptoxanthin and zinc has stimulatory effects on gene expression, protein synthesis, and cell proliferation in osteoblastic cells in rat femoral tissues. This may contribute to their enhancing effect on bone components in femoral tissues of rats *in vivo*.

The combination of β-cryptoxanthin plus zinc at a lower concentration has a synergistic effect on bone components *in vivo*. The combination of β-cryptoxanthin plus zinc has potentiality in the prevention of bone loss with aging. This finding is interested in respect of the development of new supplement with the composition of food factors that reveal a potent-anabolic effect in prevention of osteoporosis. Also, it would be useful to identify some of the foods that contain higher levels of β-cryptoxanthin and zinc.

Treatment of Bone Loss with Intake with Dietaryβ-Cryptoxanthin

As mentioned above, β-cryptoxanthin has been shown to have stimulatory effects on osteoblastic bone formation and suppressive effects on osteoclastic bone resorption *in vitro*. The preventive effect of β-cryptoxanthin on osteoporosis has been demonstrated using animal models.

β-Cryptoxanthin Reveals an Anabolic Effect on Bone in Young and Aged Rats

The anabolic effects of β-cryptoxanthin on bone components in young and aged rats have been examined.β-Cryptoxanthin (100, 250, or 500 μg/kg body weight) was orally administered once daily for 7 days to young male rats [264]. The administration of β-cryptoxanthin (250, or 500 μg/kg) caused a significant increase in alkaline phosphatase activity, DNA and calcium contents in the femoral-diaphyseal and -metaphyseal tissues [265]. Such an effect was also observed in the femoral tissues of aged (50-week-old) female rats [266]. β-Cryptoxanthin has been shown to have an anabolic effect on bone components in rats *in vivo*.

β-Cryptoxanthin Prevents Bone Loss Induced in Diabetic Rats

β-Cryptoxanthin has been sown to have preventive effects on bone loss in the pathophysiologic states. Bone loss is induced in streoptozotocin (STZ)-diabetic rats [266]. Young rats received a single subcutaneous administration of STZ (60 mg/kg body weight), and then the animals were orally administered β-cryptoxanthin (50 or 100 μg/kg) once daily for 7 or 14 days. The administration of STZ caused a significant decrease in body weight and a significant increase in serum glucose, triglyceride, and calcium levels, indicating a diabetic state [266]. These alterations were prevented after the administration of β-cryptoxanthin (50 or 100 μg/kg) for 14 days [266]. Alkaline phosphatase activity, DNA and calcium contents in the femoral-diaphyseal and -metaphyseal tissues were significantly decreased in STZ-diabetic rats [266]. These decreases were prevented after the administration of β-cryptoxanthin (50 or 100 μg/kg) for 14 days [266]. Thus, the intake of β-cryptoxanthin has been found to have preventive effects on STZ-diabetic state and bone loss in STZ-diabetic rats.

β-Cryptoxanthin Prevents Bone Loss in Ovariectomized Rats

Bone loss is induced after ovriectomy (OVX), which is a model of postmenopausal osteoporosis. The effect of β-cryptoxanthin on OVX-induced bone loss has been examined [267]. β-Cryptoxanthin (50 or 100 μg/kg body weight) was orally administered once daily for 3 months to OVX rats. The analysis using peripheral quantitative computed tomography shows that OVX induced a significant decrease in mineral content and mineral density in the femoral-diaphyseal and -metaphyseal tissues [267]. These decreases were significantly prevented after the administration of β-cryptoxanthin (50 or 100 μg/kg). Moreover, OVX induced a significant decrease in bone biochemical components. These decreases were completely prevented after the administration of β-cryptoxanthin (50 or 100 μg/kg). β-Cryptoxanthin has been found to have preventive effects on OVX-induced bone loss *in vivo* [267].

Intake of Dietary β-Cryptoxanthin Reveals a Treatment Effect in Menopausal Women

The effects of β-cryptoxanthin on bone metabolism in human have been investigated using serum bone metabolic markers. Serum bone-specific alkaline phosphatase and γ-carboxylated osteocalcin are bone metabolic markers of osteoblastic bone formation [268, 269]. Serum bone TRACP and N-telopeptides of type I collagen are metabolic markers of osteoclastic bone resorption [270, 271]. The effects of prolonged intake of juice prepared from Satsuma mandarin (*Citrus unshiu* MARC) containing β-cryptoxanthin on circulating biochemical markers of bone metabolism in human subjects, including menopausal woman, has been examined [272 - 274].

Effect of β-cryptoxanthin Intake in Healthy Human Subjects

Twenty-one volunteers (10 males and 11 females) were divided into two groups of ten volunteers (5 males and 5 females) and eleven volunteers (5 males and 6 females), and each group was given sequentially juice (192 ml) containing two different contents of β-cryptoxanthin once a day for 28 or 56 days as follows: either regular juice with naturally occurring 802 μgβ-cryptoxanthin/100 ml or a reinforced juice containing 1500 μgβ-cryptoxanthin/100 ml [272].

The intake of regular juice for 28 or 56 days in healthy subjects caused a significant increase in serum γ-carboxylated osteocalcin concentration, and the intake for 56 days produces a significant decrease in serum bone TRACP activity [272]. Moreover, the intake of theβ-cyptoxanthin reinforced juice for 28 or 56 days caused a significant increase in serum γ-carboxylated osteocalcin concentration and a corresponding decrease in serum bone TRACP activity and *N*-telopeptide of type I collagen [272]. These findings suggest that the intake ofβ-cyptoxanthin reinforced juice has a stimulatory effect on osteoblastic bone formation and inhibitory effect on osteoclastic bone resorption in normal individuals [272].

Serumβ-cyptoxanthin concentration was significantly increased after the intake of regular juice for 56 days [273]. This increase was enhanced after the intake ofβ-cyptoxanthin-reinforced juice. The intake of regular juice or ofβ-cyptoxanthin-reinforced juice for 56 days caused a significant increase in serum γ-carboxylated osteocalcin and a significant decrease in serum bone TRACP activity [273]. A possible relationship between serumβ-cyptoxanthin and circulating γ-carboxylated osteocalcin concentrations was found by using the value obtained from all groups for before intake and with the intake of regular juice andβ-cyptoxanthin-reinforced juice. A negative relationship between serumβ-cyptoxanthin concentation and circulating TRACP activity was observed [273].

This study shows that a relationship between serum β-cyptoxanthin and circulating bone metabolic markers is found in healthy individuals with the intake of juice containing β-cyptoxanthin.

Effect of β-cryptoxanthin Intake in Menopausal Women

Ninety volunteers, aged 27-65 years (19 men and 71 women), were enrolled in this study [274]. The seventy-one females included 35 premenopausal women (ages, 27-50 years) and 36 menopausal women (ages, 46-65 years). Volunteers were divided into four groups; placebo juice without β-cyptoxanthin (5 men and 19 women), juice containing β-cyptoxanthin at 1.5 mg/200 ml of juice/day (4 men and 17 women), 3.0 mg/day (5 men and 17 women), and 6.0 mg/day (5 men and 18 women). Placebo or juice (200 ml) was ingested once a day for 28 or 56 days.

Serum β-cryptoxanthin concentrations were significantly increased after the intake of juice containing β-cryptoxanthin (1.5, 3.0, or 6.0 mg/day) for 28 or 56 days, and the increases were dose-dependent [273]. A significant increase in serumβ-cryptoxanthin concentration was also observed at 28 days at the end of intake, indicating that the carotenoid is stable in the serum. Serumβ-cryptoxanthin concentration was in the range of 4.20 x 10^{-7} M to 4.89 x 10^{-7} M in the placebo groups. The intake of juice reinforced withβ-cryptoxanthin concentration at doses of 1.5, 3.0, or 6.0 mg/day significantly increased the serum concentration to 2.43 x 10^{-6},

4.06 x 10^{-6}, or 5.38 x 10^{-6} M, respectively [274]. These increases were about 5 or 10 fold as compared with the value obtained before intake or after placebo intake. It has been shown that the serum concentration of β-cryptoxanthin increased due to the consumption of vegetable juice in women from 1.3 x 10^{-7} to 5.3 x 10^{-7} M [249].

In ninety volunteers (aged 27-65 years), serum bone-specific alkaline phosphatase activity was significantly increased after the intake of juice containing β-cryptoxanthin (3.0 or 6.0 mg/day) for 56 days as compared with the value obtained before intake [274]. Serum γ-carboxylated osteocalcin concentration was increased after the intake of juice containing β-cryptoxanthin (3.0 or 6.0 mg/day) for 28 or 56 days as compared with the value obtained before intake or after the intake of placebo juice [274]. Serum TRACP activity and type I collagen *N*-telopeptide concentration were decreased after the intake of juice containing β-cryptoxanthin (3.0 or 6.0 mg/day) for 28 or 56 days as compared with the value obtained before intake or after intake of placebo juice, and significant decreases were also seen after the intake of 1.5 mg/dayβ-cryptoxanthin as compared with the value obtained before intake [274].

In menopausal women (36 volunteers), bone-specific alkaline phosphatase activity and γ-carboxylated osteocalcin concentration were significantly increased after the intake of juice containing β-cryptoxanthin (3.0 or 6.0 mg/day) for 56 days as compared with the value obtained after placebo intake [274]. Also, this intake caused a significant decrease in bone TRACP activity and type I collagen *N*-telopeptide concentration. Thus, prolonged intake of β-cryptoxanthin-reinforced juice has been demonstrated to have stimulatory effects on osteoblastic bone formation and inhibitory effects on osteoclastic bone resorption in menopausal women.

Meanwhile, serum calcium, inorganic phosphorus, and parathyroid hormone (intact) were not changed after the intake of β-cryptoxanthin-containing juice for 28 or 56 days. Other serum biochemical findings were not changed after the intake of juice containing β-cryptoxanthin (3.0 or 6.0 mg/day) for 56 days. The safety of β-cryptoxanthin in human is confirmed [274].

As mentioned above, the intake of juice reinforced withβ-cryptoxanthin (3.0 or 6.0 mg/day) has been found to have a significant effect on circulating bone metabolic markers in men, premenopausal women, and menopausal women [274]. This indicates that the effects ofβ-cryptoxanthin in stimulating bone formation and inhibiting bone resorption are present in both sexes. Interstingly, the intake of juice reinforced withβ-cryptoxanthin (3.0 or 6.0 mg/day) has been found to have effects on circulating bone metabolic markers in menopausal women, indicating that the supplementation ofβ-cryptoxanthin has preventive effects on bone loss due to osteoporosis in menopausal women. This preventive effect is obvious at a dose ofβ-cryptoxanthin of 3.0 mg/day in menopausal women. This dose may be suitable in the prevention of osteoporosis in human subjects.

Thus, the intake of reinforced juice, which contains moreβ-cryptoxanthin than regular juice, has been demonstrated to have a preventive effect on bone loss that accompanies an increase in age.

β-Cryptoxanthin and Bone Health: Epidemiological Evidence

On the based on our findings, it has been shown that epidemiological studies show that the intakes of fruit and vegetables containingβ-cryptoxanthin may reduce the risk of osteoporosis [275-277].

The effect of dietary antioxidants on knee structure in a cohort of healthy, middle-aged subjects with no clinical knee osteoarthritis is reported [275]. Two hundred and ninety-three healthy adults (mean age = 58.0 years) without knee pain or knee injury were selected from an existing community-based cohort. The intake of antioxidant vitamins and food sources by these individuals was estimated from a food frequency questionnaire at baseline. The cartilage volume, bone area, cartilage defects and bone marrow lesions were assessed approximately 10 years later using magnetic resonance imaging. Higher vitamin C intake was associated with a reduced risk of bone marrow lesions and with a reduction in the tibial plateau bone area. There was an inverse association between fruit intake and the tibial plateau bone area and between fruit intake and the risk of bone marrow lesions. Neither fruit intake nor vitamin C intake was significantly associated with the cartilage volume or cartilage defects.

Lutein and zeaxanthin intake was associated with a decreased risk of cartilage defects, and vitamin E intake tended top be positively associated with the tibial plateau bone were only after adjusting for vitamin C intake. Theβ-cryptoxanthin intake was inversely associated with the tibial plateau bone area after adjusting for vitamin E intake. These observations suggest a beneficial effect of fruit consumption and vitamin C intake as they are associated with a reduction in bone size and the number of bone marrow lesions, both of which are important in the pathogenesis of knee osteoarthritis [275].

Bone mineral density (BMD) in post-menopausal female subjects has been shown to associate with serum antioxidant carotenoids. A total of six hundred ninety-nine subjects (222 males and 477 females) who had received health examinations in the town of Mikkabi, Shizuoka Prefecture, Japan, participated in the study [276]. Radial BMD was measured using dual-energy X-ray absorptiometry. The associations of serum carotenoid concentrations with the dadial BMD were evaluated cross-sectionally. In male and pre-menopausal female subjects, the six serum carotenoids were not associated with the radial BMD. On the other hand, in post-menopausal female subjects, serumβ-cryptoxanthin and β-carotene were weakly but positively correlated with the radial BMD. After adjustment for confounders, the odds ratio (OR) for the lowest quartile of BMD in the high groups of serum β-cryptoxanthin against the lowest quartile was 0.45 in post-menopausal female subjects. However, this association was not significant after further adjusting for intakes of minerals and vitamins. Antioxidant carotenoids, especiallyβ-cryptoxanthin, significantly but partly associated with the radial BMD in post-menopausal female subjects [276].

Moreover, epidemiological studies showed that high intakes of carotenoids might be useful to maintain bone health [277]. A follow-up on 146 male and 99 pre- and 212 post-menopausal female subjects from the Mikkabi study, Shizuoka, Japan, was conducted [277]. Those who participated in previous BMD surveys and completed four years of follow-up were examined longitudinally. During a 4-year follow-up, 15 of the post-menopausal female subjects developed new-onset osteoporosis. In contrast, none of the male and pre-menopausal female subjects did. In male and pre-menopausal female subjects, the six serum carotenoids at the baseline were not associated with bone loss. On the other hand, in post-menopausal female subjects, the 4-year bone loss of radius was inversely associated with the serum carotenoid concentrations, especially in β-carotene. After adjustments for confounders, the odds ratios (OR) for osteoporosis in the highest tertiles of serum β-carotene and β-cryptoxanthin against the lowest tertiles were 0.24 (95% confidence interval 0.05-1.21) and 0.07 (CI: 0.01-0.88), respectively. Serum β-cryptoxanthin was also inversely associated with the risk for osteopenia and/or osteoporosis (P for trend, 0.037). In addition, this retrospective analysis revealed that subjects who developed osteoporosis and/or osteopenia during the survey period had significantly lower serum concentrations of β-cryptoxanthin and β-carotene at the baseline than those in the normal group. Thus, antioxidant carotenoids, especially β-cryptoxanthin and β-carotene, have been found to be inversely associated with the change of radial BMD in post-menopausal female subjects.

Interestingly, seasonal variation of serum α- and β-cryptoxanthin and 25-OH-vitamin D_3 in women with osteoporosis has been examined [278]. In six hundred fourty-four women with osteoporosis, serum β-cryptoxanthin and 25-OH-vitamin D_3 showed a weak but significant correlation and exhibited a complementary seasonal distribution [278]. Dietary intake and serum levels ofβ-cryptoxanthin have been inversely related to different bone and joint disorders and in vitro and animal studies have shown thatβ-cryptoxanthin displays a unique anabolic effect on bone calcification. Due to the emerging role of β-cryptoxanthin in bone biology, this study was aimed to assess the serum distribution and variability ofβ-cryptoxanthin and their potential relation to 25-OH-vitamin D_3 in women with osteoporosis [278].

Overall, significant seasonal variations were found for the three analyses and inter-individual variation was also high (60-73%).β-Cryptoxanthin and 25-OH- vitamin D_3 exhibited a marked complementary seasonal distribution in serum, with vitamin D displaying the highest values in summer andβ-cryptoxanthin in winter.

Given the anabolic effect ofβ-cryptoxanthin on bone calcification and its complementary seasonal distribution with respect to 25-OH- vitamin D_3, the potential role of β-cryptoxanthin as a sustainable nutritional approach to improving bone health deserves to be further evaluated [278].

Dietary Total Carotenoids and Osteoporosis Prevention

In vitro and *in vivo* studies suggest that carotenoids may stimulate bone formation and may inhibit bone resorption. The associations of total and individual carotenoid intake (α-carotene, β-carotene, β-cryptoxanthin, lycopene, lutein and zeaxanthin) with incident hip fracture and nonvertebral osteoporotic fracture are shown [279]. Three hundred seventy men and 576 women (mean age, 75 ± 5 years) from the Framingham Osteoporosis Study completed a food frequency questionnaire (FFQ) in 1988–1989 and were followed for hip fracture until 2005 and nonvertebral fracture until 2003. Tertiles of carotenoid intake were created from estimates obtained using the Willett FFQ adjusting for total energy (residual method). HRs were estimated using Cox-proportional hazards regression, adjusting for sex, age, body mass index, height, total energy, calcium and vitamin D intake, physical activity, alcohol, smoking, multivitamin use, and current estrogen use. A total of 100 hip fractures occurred over 17 years of follow-up. Subjects in the highest textile of total carotenoid intake had lower risk of hip fracture. Subjects with higher lycopene intake had lower risk of hip fracture and nonvertebral fracture. A weak protective trend was observed for total β-carotene for hip fracture alone, but associations do not reach statistical significance. No significant associations are observed with α-carotene, β-cryptoxanthin, or lutein plus zeaxanthin. These findings suggest a protective role of several carotenoids for bone health in older adults [279].

Antioxidant defenses may be compromised in osteoporotic women. Little is known about fruit and vegetable or carotenoid consumption among postmenopausal women. The primary carotenoids in human serum are α- and β-carotene, lycopene, β-cryptoxanthin, lutein and zeaxanthin [280]. The interrelationships among serum carotenoid concentrations, fruit and vegetable intake, and osteoporosis in postmenopausal women (n = 59, 62.7 +/- 8.8 years) are shown [280]. Bone density was assessed by dual energy x-ray absorptiometry (DEXA) and osteoporosis diagnosis was based upon T-scores. Serum samples (n = 53) and three-day diet records (n = 49) were analyzed. Logistic regression analyzed differences between carotenoids after adjusting for serum retinol; supplement usage; milk, yogurt, fruit, and vegetable intake; and body mass index. Pearson statistics correlated carotenoids with specific fruit or vegetable intake. Serum lycopene concentrations were lower in the osteoporosis group than controls. The intake of β-cryptoxanthin was higher in the osteoporosis group. Total fruit and vegetable intakes were correlated with serum lycopene and β-cryptoxanthin [280].

Recent studies have showed that antioxidants may reduce the risk of osteoporosis. The associations of BMD with dietary patterns of antioxidant vitamins and carotenoids are shown [281]. A total of 293 post-menopausal female subjects who had received health examinations in the town of Mikkabi, Shizuoka Prefecture, Japan, is participated in the study [281]. Radial BMD was measured using DEXA. Dietary patterns were identified on a selected set of antioxidants through principal component factor analysis. Three dietary patterns are identified. The "retinol" pattern, characterized by notably high intakes of preformed retinol, zeaxanthin, and vitamin E, is positively associated with the risk for low BMD [281].

In contrast, the "β-cryptoxanthin" pattern, characterized by notably high intakes of β-cryptoxanthin and vitamin C, is negatively associated with low BMD [281]. The odds ratios for low BMD in the highest tertiles of dietary intakes of preformed retinol, vitamin C, and β-cryptoxanthin against the lowest tertiles are 3.22 [95% confidence interval (CI), 1.38-7.51], 0.25 (CI, 0.10-0.66), and 0.40 (CI, 0.17-0.92), respectively, after adjustments for confounders [281]. However, negative associations of vitamin C and β-cryptoxanthin with low BMD were not significant after further adjustment for intake of β-cryptoxanthin or vitamin C, respectively [281]. Higher intakes of both vitamin C and β-cryptoxanthin were significantly associated with low BMD [281]. The findings suggest the combination of vitamin C and β-cryptoxanthin intakes might provide benefit to bone health in post-menopausal Japanese female subjects. The combination of vitamin C and β-cryptoxanthin may be associated with radial BMD in post-menopausal women.

It is possible that the preventive effect of β-cryptoxanthin on osteoporosis is enhanced with other carotenoids and factors in foods. This may be important in maintaining bone health in human life with food intake.

Conclusion

Among various carotenoids, β-cryptoxanthin, which is abundant in Satsuma mandarin orange (*Citrus unshiu* MARC.), has a unique anabolic effect on bone mass due to stimulating osteoblastic bone formation and inhibiting osteoclastic bone resorption. β-Cryptoxanthin modulates gene expression of various proteins that involve in bone formation in osteoblasts and bone resorption in osteoclasts. The intake of dietaryβ-cryptoxanthin has been shown to have preventive effects on bone loss in animal models for osteoporosis and restorative effects on bone metabolism in menopausal women. The role of β-cryptoxanthin in bone health has been also shown in human subjects with epidemiological studies. β-Cryptoxanthin may have an important role in the prevention and treatment of osteoporosis. In addition, the intake of foods that contain β-cryptoxanthin and other carotenoids may have a role in maintaining bone health and decrease in bone loss. The supplemental intake of β-cryptoxanthin with higher dose may have a pharmacologic role in the therapy of osteoporosis. Clinical studies usingβ-cryptoxanthin will be expected in the development of new drug for osteoporosis therapy.

Chapter 7

Plant Bioactive Factor *P*-Hydroxycinnamic Acid and Bone Homeostasis: Role in Osteoporosis Treatment

Chemical compounds in food and plants, which regulate bone homeostasis, have been to be worthy of notice in maintaining bone health and in the prevention and treatment of bone loss with increasing age. It appears increasingly likely that as-yet-unidentified factors found in the daily consumption of fruits or vegetables may play a role in the building of optimal peak bone mass and in the preservation of decreased bone mass with aging. Cinnamic acid is present in many plant and fruits. Among of cinnamic acid, *p*-hydroxycinnamic acid (HCA), ferulic acid, caffeic acid, or 3,4-dimethoxycinnamic acid, HCA was uniquely found to have a potential-anabolic effect on bone mineralization *in vitro*. HCA is an intermediate-metabolic substance in plants and fruits and is synthesized from tyrosine. HCA stimulates osteoblastic bone formation and suppresses osteoclastic bone resorption *in vitro*. Oral administration of HCA was found to have a preventive effect on bone loss induced with ovarietomy and diabetic state. Thus, HCA may have an effect in the prevention and treatment of osteoporosis. This chapter has been written to outline the recent advances concerning the role of HCA in the regulation of bone homeostasis and in the treatment of osteoporosis.

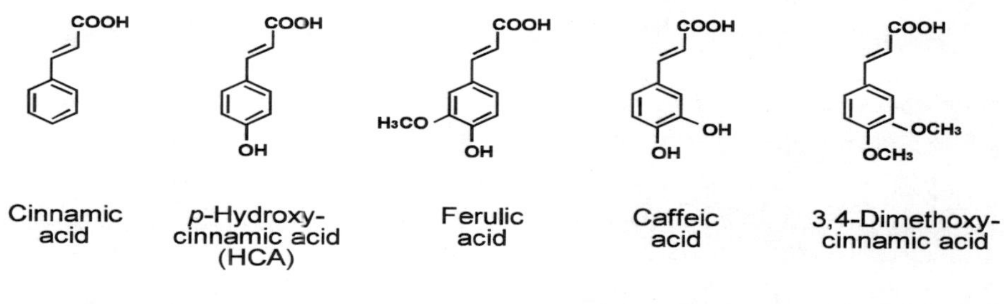

Figure 18. Chemical structures of cinnamic acid and its related compounds. The molecular weight of cinnamic acid, *p*-hydroxycinnamic acid (HCA), ferulic acid, caffeic acid, and 3, 4-dimethoxycinnamic acid (DCA) is 148.2, 164.2, 194.2, 180.2, and 208.3, respectively. Among of these compounds, HCA has been shown to have an anabolic effect on bone.

HCA Stimulates Osteoblastogenesis *In Vitro*

The effects of cinnamic acid or its related compounds on bone mineralization have been examined using rat femoral tissues *in vitro* [282]. These chemical structures are shown in Figure 18. The effects of cinnamic acid and its related compounds on bone mineralization have not been determined so far. Then, the rat femoral-diaphyseal or -metaphyseal tissues were cultured for 48 hours in a medium containing cinnamic acid, HCA, ferulic acid, caffeic acid, or 3,4-dimethoxycinnamic acid *in vitro* [282]. Culture with HCA (10^{-5} or 10^{-4} M) caused an increase in calcium content in the diaphyseal and metaphyseal tissues [282]. This effect was not observed after culture with cinnamic acid or other compounds at the concentration of 10^{-5} or 10^{-4} M. In addition, alkaline phosphatase activity and DNA content in the diaphyseal or metaphyseal tissues was also increased after culture with HCA (10^{-5} or 10^{-4} M) [282]. The effects of HCA (10^{-4} M) in increasing alkaline phosphatase activity, DNA and calcium contents in the diaphyseal or metaphyseal tissues were completely depressed in the presence of cycloheximide (10^{-6} M), an inhibitor of protein synthesis. Thus, HCA has been found to have a unique-anabolic effect on bone metabolism, which results from newly synthesized protein components [282]. DNA content in the bone tissues may be partly involved in the number of bone cells including osteoblasts, osteocytes, and osteoclasts. HCA increased DNA content in the femoral-diaphyseal and -metaphyseal tissues of rats *in vitro* and stimulated bone mineralization. HCA may stimulate proliferation of osteoblastic cells in the bone tissues *in vitro* and has a stimulatory effect on bone formation.

HCA is hydroxylated at 4-position of cinnamic acid in the chemical structure of cinnamic acid and its related compounds as shown in Figure 18. This chemical form may have an anabolic effect on bone metabolism, suggesting a relationship of structure and activity of cinnamic acid.

HCA has been found to stimulate osteoblastogenesis. Osteoblastic MC3T3-E1 cells *in vitro* were cultured for 72 hours in a minimum essential medium containing 10% fetal bovine serum (FBS) and the subconfluent cells were changed to a medium containing either vehicle or HCA (10^{-7} to 10^{-5} M) without FBS [283]. Culture with HCA (10^{-7} to 10^{-5} M) did not have a significant effect on cell proliferation of osteoblastic cells in reaching subconfluent monolayers [283]. Also, the number of osteoblastic cells after reaching to subconfluent was not changed after culture with HCA, indicating that the compound does not induce cell death [283]. However, culture with HCA caused an increase in DNA content in osteoblastic cells [283]. The effect of HCA in increasing DNA content in osteoblastic cells was also seen in the absence of FBS [283]. HCA may have a stimulatory effect on DNA synthesis in osteoblastic cells.

Alkaline phosphatase is involved in mineralization in osteoblastic cells. Alkaline phosphatase activity in osteoblastic cells was significantly increased after culture with HCA (10^{-7} to 10^{-5} M) for 24 - 72 hours [283], indicating that HCA stimulates the differentiation in osteoblastic cells. The results of Alizarin red stain showed that the prolonged culture with HCA markedly stimulates mineralization in osteoblastic cells; mineralization was stimulated after culture with HCA (10^{-8} to 10^{-5} M) for 7, 14, or 21 days [283]. This finding support the view that culture with HCA stimulates the differentiation of osteoblastic cells and that promotes mineralization in the cells. In addition, HCA caused a significant increase in calcium content in rat femoral tissue culture *in vitro*. HCA has stimulatory effects on osteoblastic differentiation and mineralization [283]. In addition, culture with HCA has been shown to have stimulatory effects on osteoblastogenesis and mineralization in mouse bone marrow culture *in vitro*.

HCA Suppresses Osteoclastogenesis *In Vitro*

Osteoclasts are generated from bone marrow stem cells. Receptor activator of the nuclear factor kappa B (NF-κB) (RANK) ligand (RANKL) plays a pivotal role in osteoclastogenesis from bone marrow cells [8, 9]. RANKL is produced from osteoblasts in response to osteoporotic factors, such as parathyroid hormone (PTH), prostaglandine E_2 (PGE_2), and 1, 25-dihydroxyvitamin D_3 [1, $25(OH)_2D_3$] [162-164]. RANKL acts osteoclast progenitors and stimulates osteoclast differentiation. Osteoclastic cells are differentiated from bone marrow stromal cells. Osteoclastogenesis is stimulated through macrophage colony-stimulating factor (M-CSF) and RANKL *in vitro* [77, 78]. A soluble fragment containing part of the extra-cellular domain of RANKL (the carboxyterminal half of the protein, amino acids 158-316) is capable of promoting osteoclastogenesis in the presence of M-CSF [77, 78]. The receptor protein RANK for RANKL is expressed on the surface of osteoclast progenitors. The interaction of RANKL with its receptor RANK leads to the recruitment of the signaling adaptor molecules TRAFs (TNF receptor-associated factors) to the receptor complex and the activation of nuclear factor-κB (NF-κB) and c-Jun N-terminal kinase (JNK) [284]. The protein kinase C family enzyme has a role in the regulation of osteoclast formation and function potentially by participating in the extracellular signal-regulated kinase (ERK) signaling pathway of M-CSF and RANKL [285-287].

HCA has been found to have a suppressive effect on bone resorption induced by bone-resorbing factors in the bone tissue culture *in vitro* [282]. PTH or 1, $25(OH)_2D_3$ is known as bone-resorbing factors [162, 163]. Culture with PTH caused a decrease in calcium content and an increase in the activity of tartrate-resistant acid phosphatase (TRACP), which is a marker enzyme in osteoclastic cells, in the diaphyseal or metaphyseal tissues and a corresponding elevation in medium glucose consumption and lactic acid production by the bone tissues [282]. These alterations were completely depressed after culture with HCA (10^{-5} or 10^{-4} M). Thus, HCA has been shown to have a suppressive effect on bone resorption in the bone tissue culture *in vitro* [282].

Culture with HCA has also been found to have suppressive effects on PTH-, prostaglandin E_2 (PGE_2)-, or tumor necrosis factor-α (TNF-α)-induced osteoclast-like cell formation from mouse bone marrow *in vitro* [288]. HCA did not have an effect on the proliferation of bone marrow cells, suggesting that the compound did not have a toxic effect on the cells [288]. The suppressive effects of HCA on osteoclast-like cell formation were remarkable at the earlier stage of the differentiation to osteoclasts in bone marrow cultures [288]. In addition, such suppressive effect of HCA was also observed at the later stage of osteoclastogenesis [288]. HCA may have an effect on the process of the differentiation from mononuclear osteoclast to osteoclast [288].

Moreover, HCA suppressed osteoclast-like cell formation induced by PTH or PGE_2 [288]. The suppressive effects of HCA were partly involved in RANKL expression and/or RANKL action, which are related to the effects of PTH and PGE_2. Culture with HCA suppressed RANKL plus M-CSF-induced osteoclast-like cell formation in mouse bone marrow culture *in vitro* [288]. Presumably, the suppressive effects of HCA are involved in RANKL expression and/or RANKL action, which are related to the effect of PTH or PGE_2.

TNF-α is an autocrine factor in osteoclasts, promoting their differentiation and mediating RANKL-induced osteoclastogenesis [284]. TNF-α has also been shown to mediate via its p55 receptor in lypoplysaccaride-stimulated osteoclastogenesis [284]. TNF-α-induced osteoclast-like cell formation in mouse bone marrow cultures was significantly suppressed after culture with HCA [288]. HCA may suppress osteoclastogenesis that is mediated through RANKL and TNF-α.

Phorbol 12-myristate 13-acetate (PMA) is an activator of protein kinase C. PMA stimulated osteoclast-like cell formation in mouse bone marrow cultures, and PMA-induced osteoclastogenesis was suppressed after culture with HCA [288]. Moreover, HCA was found to have a suppressive effect on dibutyryl cyclic AMP-induced osteoclast-like cell formation in mouse bone marrow cultures [288]. The activation of the protein kinase C- or protein kinase A may be related to RANKL signaling in osteoclastogeneasis. HCA may have a suppressive effect on osteoclastogenesis that is mediated through signaling mechanim of protein kinase C or protein kinase A. Culture with HCA caused an inhibition of RANKL plus M-CSF-induced osteoclast-like cell formation in mouse bone marrow culture *in vitro* [288]. This observation may support the view that HCA represses the binding of RANKL to receptor RANK and that suppresses RANKL signaling in osteoclastogenesis.

The effect of HCA in inhibiting RANKL plus M-CSF-induced osteoclastogenesis was completely depressed in the presence of cycloheximide, an inhibitor of protein synthesis in the translational processes [288]. The stimulatory effect of RANKL plus M-CSF on osteoclastogenesis was not suppressed in the presence of cycloheximide or 5,6-dichloro-1-β-D-ribofuranosylbenzimidazole (DRB), an inhibitor of transcriptional processes [288]. The suppressive effect of HCA on osteoclastogenesis may be partly involved in newly synthesized protein components, which induce suppressor protein. HCA may have effects on the expression of osteoprotegerin (OPG), which is a regulator of osteoclast differentiation [77, 78], in osteoblasts. This remains to be determined.

HCA Stimulates Osteoblastogenesis and Suppresses Osteoclastogenesis Through Suppression of NF-KB Activation

The NF-κB signal transduction pathway has long been recognized as critical for osteoclast development and function [29, 30] and double knockout of p50 and p52 NF-κB subunits leads to osteopetrosis due to a severe defect in osteoclast differentiation in these mice [289, 290]. Furthermore, it has been reported that NF-κB signaling represses basal osteoblast differentiation and mineralization in MC3T3 cells and antagonizes TGF-β1 and BMP-2 mediated MC3T3 mineralization by downregulating Smad activation [290]. Other studies have found that NF-κB signaling antagonizes Smad activation in Saos2 osteosarcoma cells by a mechanism involving induction of inhibitory Smad7 [290, 291].

TNF-α is an inflammatory cytokine that antagonizes bone formation *in vivo* and osteoblastic differentiation *in vitro* [289, 290]. These effects are mediated in large measure through NF-κB signaling. Inflammatory levels of TNF-α are known to impact bone formation; however, it has been recently reported that basal TNF-α levels *in vivo* also dramatically lower the basal bone formation rate [290]. HCA may promote accumulation of basal bone mass, and forestall bone loss during osteoporotic states, in part by antagonizing TNF-α-induced NF-κB. Interestingly, HCA prevented TNF-α-induced suppression of mineralization in osteoblastic 3T3-E1 cells and repressed TNF-α-induced NF-κB activation in osteoblastic cells [292, 293]. Culture with HCA was also found to suppress the differentiation of preosteoclasts (RAW267.4 cells) to osteoclasts induced by RANKL through suppression of NF-κB activation [293].

The 5 members of the mammalian NF-κB family RelA/p65, RelB, c-Rel, NF-κB1/p50, and NF-κB2/p52 are activated through one of two specific pathways, the canonical NF-κB pathway or an alternative pathway [294]. In the canonical pathway, activation of the inhibitor of IκB kinase (IKK) complex leads to phosphorylation of the NF-κB-associated IκBα, catalyzing its ubiquitination and proteasomal degradation, and in the process releasing active NF-κB dimmers that translocate to the nucleus and enhance the transcription of target genes [294]. In the alternative NF-κB pathway, NF-κB-inducing kinase (NIK) and IKKα target p100 for proteolytic processing, thereby releasing active RelB-containing dimmers [294]. Differential regulation of these two pathways by HCA could provide a more detail explanation for the suppressive effect observed in TNF-α-induced NF-κB activation.

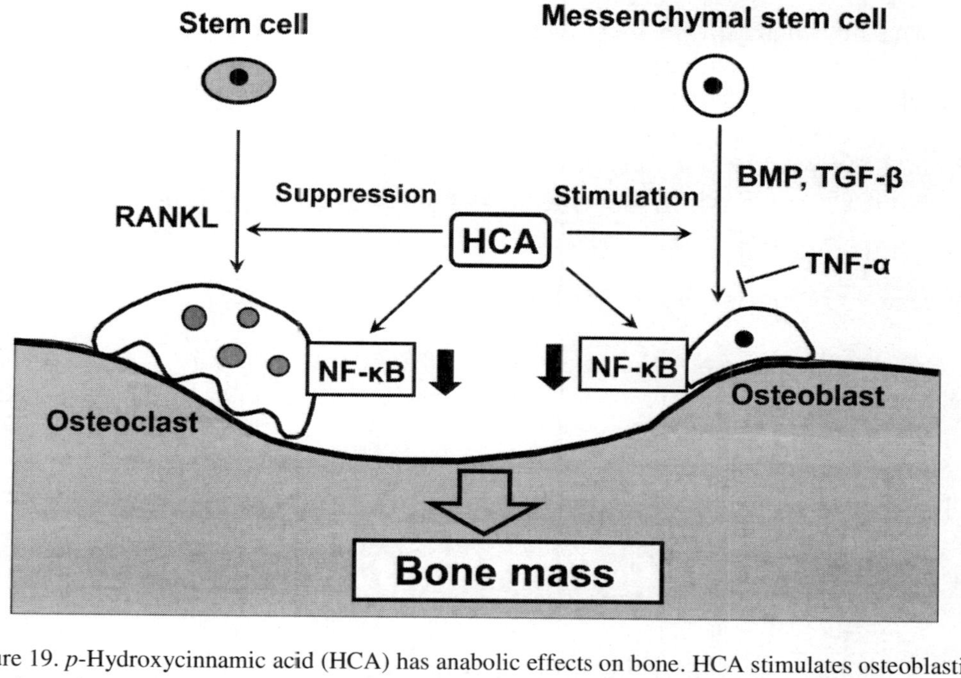

Figure 19. *p*-Hydroxycinnamic acid (HCA) has anabolic effects on bone. HCA stimulates osteoblastic bone formation and suppresses osteoclastic bone resorption, thereby increasing bone mass. The osteogenic effect of HCA is mediated through the suppression of NF-κB activation.

The cellular mechanism by which HCA stimulates osteoblastic bone formation and suppresses osteoclastic bone resorption is mediated through the suppression of NF-κB activation as shown in Figure 19.

HCA Treats Osteoporosis *In Vivo*

HCA Has Anabolic Effects on Bone

The anabolic effects of HCA on the bone of rats *in vivo* have been shown [35-37]. Rats were orally administered HCA (10, 20, or 50 mg/ kg body weight) once daily for seven days [35]. The administration of HCA did not cause a significant change in body weight or serum calcium and inorganic phosphorus levels. Alkaline phosphatase activity, DNA and calcium contents in the diaphyseal and metaphyseal tissues were increased after the administration of HCA (20 or 50 mg/kg) [295]. Diaphyseal calcium and metaphyseal DNA contents were increased with the dose of HCA 10 mg/kg. These findings suggest that oral administration of HCA induces anabolic effects on bone mineralization in normal growing rats.

The activity of TRACP, which is a marker enzyme of osteoclastic bone resorption, is enhanced by bone-resorbing factors [296]. Oral administration of HCA (10, 20, or 50 mg/kg) caused a significant decrease in TRACP activity in the femoral-diaphyseal and –metaphyseal tissues of rats [295]. This suggests that the administration of HCA induces a decrease in bone-resorbing activity in the femoral tissues of rats *in vivo*.

The mixture of phenolic acids found in the serum of young rats fed blueberries has been reported to stimulate osteoblast differentiation, resulting in significantly increased bone mass [297]. Greater bone formation in blueberries diet-fed animals is associated with increase in osteoblast progenitors and osteoblast differentiation and reduced osteoclastogenesis [297]. The most of the phenolic acids in the circulation of blueberries diet-fed animals are either metabolites or breakdown products of polyphenols and phenolic acids found in blueberries [39]. Interestingly, HCA is found in the serum after diet of blueberries [297].

HCA Prevents Ovariectomy-induced Bone Loss

The preventive effect of HCA on osteoporosis has been examined using ovariectomized (OVX) rats, an animal model for osteoporosis [298]. HCA (0.25 or 0.5 mg/kg body weight) was orally administered once daily for 30 days to OVX rats. The analysis using a peripheral quantitative computed tomography (pQCT) showed that OVX caused bone loss in the femoral-metaphyseal tissues [298]. Such bone loss was restored after the administration of HCA (2.5 or 5 mg/kg body weight) to OVX rats [298]. Mineral content, mineral density and polar strength strain index in the femoral-metaphyseal tissues were decreased in OVX rats [298]. These decreases were restored after the administration of HCA (5 mg/kg) to OVX rats [298]. Especially, the polar stress strain index is an indicator of bone strength. Moreover, OVX caused a decrease in calcium content or alkaline phosphatase activity in the femoral-diaphyseal and -metaphyseal tissues. These decreases were also restored after the administration of HCA (2.5 or 5 mg/kg) to OVX rats [298]. These observations suggest that the oral administration of HCA causes a functional change in the bone of OVX rats. Thus, HCA has been shown to have preventive effects on OVX-induced bone loss of rats *in vivo*. Presumably, HCA stimulates osteoblastic bone formation and inhibits osteoclastic bone resorption *in vivo*, thereby increasing bone mass in OVX rats.

The dose with HCA 2.5 or 5 mg/kg body weight had preventive effects on the decrease in alakaline phosphatase activity and calcium content or the increase in DNA content in the femoral-diaphyseal tissues of OVX rats, although the dose of HCA 5 mg/kg had great potential effects in the restoration of OVX-induced bone change [298]. This suggests that the intake of HCA less than 2.5 mg/day/kg body weight has preventive effects on bone loss. The amount of intake of HCA in fruit and vegetables is unknown. However, the dietary intake of phytocomponent HCA may have a role in the prevention of bone loss with aging. HCA may have a preventive effect on bone loss with increasing age.

HCA Prevents Diabetic State-induced Bone Loss

Bone loss is induced in the diabetic state [299, 300]. Streptozotocin (STZ) induces type I diabetes. The preventive effects of HCA on bone loss induced in STZ-diabetic rats have been examined *in vivo* [301]. Rats received a single subcutaneous administration of STZ (60 mg/kg body weight), and then the animals were orally administered HCA (2.5, 5, or 10 mg/kg) once daily for 14 days. STZ administration caused a decrease in body weight and a significant increase in serum glucose, triglyceride and calcium levels, indicating a diabetic state [301]. These alterations were prevented after the administration of HCA (2.5, 5, or 10 mg/kg) [301]. This was a novel finding. The intake of HCA has a restorative effect on serum biochemical findings that are involved in diabetes *in vivo*. HCA may have a role in the prevention of diabetic states.

Serum calcium concentration was found to increase in STZ-diabetic rats [301]. Intestinal calcium absorption has been shown to be impaired in the diabetic state [302]. The increase in serum calcium concentration in STZ-diabetic rats may result from the release of calcium from the bone tissues; the femoral calcium content was found to markedly decrease in STZ-diabetic rats [302]. Oral administration of HCA in the diabetic rats had a significant preventive effect on hypercalcemia and bone calcium loss in the diabetic state. Thus, the intake of HCA may have a preventive effect on bone resorption in diabetic rats.

Calcium content in the femoral-diaphyseal and -metaphyseal tissues was decreased in STZ-diabetic rats [301]. Also, this decrease was prevented after oral administration of HCA (2.5, 5, or 10 mg/kg) [301]. The intake of dietary HCA may have a restorative effect on bone loss in diabetic state. Alkaline phosphatase activity in the diaphyseal and metaphyseal tissues was decreased in STZ-diabetic rats [301]. The decrease in diaphyseal alkaline phosphatase activity in STZ-diabetic rats was restored after administration of HCA (5 and 10 mg/kg). This enzyme participates in osteoblastic mineralization. The femoral alkaline phosphatase activity was decreased in diabetic rats, suggesting that osteoblastic bone mineralization is impaired in the diabetic state.

In addition, the diaphyseal DNA content was also decreased in STZ-diabetic rats [301]. The administration of HCA (2.5, 5, or 10 mg/kg) caused an increase in DNA content in the diaphyseal and metaphyseal tissues in STZ-diabetic rats [301]. DNA content in the bone tissues is an index of the number of existing bone cells [6]. HCA may stimulate an increase in bone cells including osteoblastic cells in the diaphyseal and metaphyseal tissues of STZ-diabetic rats *in vivo*. This may be partly contributed to the increase in bone calcium content in STZ-diabetic rats. Presumably, the intake of HCA has a stimulatory effect on osteoblastic bone formation in diabetic state.

Thus, the intake of HCA has a preventive effect on bone loss in STZ-diabetic rats and has a restorative effect on serum biochemical findings in the diabetic state, suggesting that HCA has a restorative effect on diabetic state. HCA may have a role in the prevention and treatment of osteoporosis in diabetic state.

Conclusion

Cinnamic acid is present in many plant and fruits. Among of cinnamic acid, *p*-hydroxycinnamic acid (HCA), ferulic acid, caffeic acid, or 3,4-dimethoxycinnamic acid, HCA has been demonstrated to have an anabolic effect on bone mass due to stimulating osteoblastic bone formation and inhibiting osteoclastic bone resorption. The action of HCA may be partly based on suppressive effects on NF-κB activation in osteoblastic cells and osteoclastic cells. The administration of HCA has a restorative effect on bone loss induced in OVX and diabetic rats. Supplemental intake of HCA may have a role in the prevention and treatment of osteoporosis.

Chapter 8

Role of Plant Flavonoid Quercetin in Osteoporosis Treatment

Flavonoid, a kind of polyphenol, possesses a fundmental chemical structure of flavone and displays yellow pigments, including flavone, isoflavon, flavonol, flavonon and quercetin, which are found in fruits, vegetables, leaves and grains. Flavonoid has a strong anti-oxidant effect.

Quercetin, a flavonol, is a plant-derived flavonoid. Its chemical structure is shown in Figure 20. It is used as an ingredient in supplements, beverages or foods. Quercetin is biosynthesized from phenylalanine. Phenylalanine is converted to 4-coumaroyl-CoA in a series of steps known as the general phenylpropanoid pathway using phenylalanine ammonia-lyase, cinnamate-4-hydroxylase, and 4-coumaroyl-CoA-ligase. 4-Coumaroyl-CoA is added to three molecules of malonyl-CoA to form tetrahydroxychalcone using 7, 2'-dihydroxy-4'-methoxyisoflavanol synthase. Tetrahydroxychalcone is then converted into naringenin using chalcone isomerase. Naringenin is then converted into eriodictyol using flavanoid 3'-hydroxylase. Eriodictyol is then converted into dihydroquercetin with flavanone 3-hydroxylase, which is then converted into quercetin using flavonol synthase. The enzyme quercitrinase can be found in *Aspergillus flavus*. Its substrates are quercitrin and H_2O and releases quercetin and L-rhamnose. It is an enzyme in the rutin catabolic pathway. Quercetin 3-O-sulfate is a human plasma quercetin metabolite.

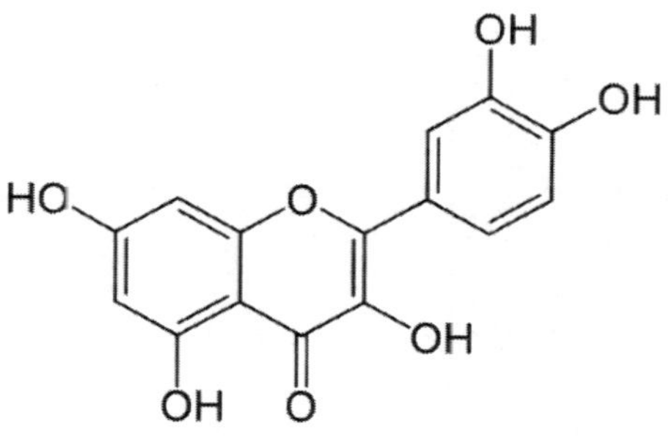

Figure 20. Chemical structure of quercetin. The molecular weight of quercetin ($C_{15}H_{10}O_7$) is 302.24.

Quercetin is the aglycone form of a number of other flavonoid glycosides, such as rutin and quercitrin, which are found in citrus fruit, buckwheat and onions. Quercetin forms the glycosides quercitrin and rutin together with rhamnose and rutinose, respectively. Likewise, guaijaverin is the 3-O-arabinoside, hyperoside is the 3-O-galactoside, isoquercitin is the 3-O-glucoside, and spiraeoside is the 4'-O-glucoside. CTN-986 is a quercetin derivative found in cottonseeds and cottonseed oil. Miquelianin is the quercetin 3-o-β-d-glucuronopyranoside.

Quercetin itself (aglycone quercetin), as opposed to quercetin glycosides, is not a normal dietary component. In a bioavailability study in rats, radiolabelled quercetin-4'-glucoside was converted to phenolic acids as it passed through the gastrointestinal tract, producing compounds not monitored in previous animal studies of aglycone quercetin. All but 4% was recovered within 72 hours (69% in urine), indicating low retention and high excretion, a characteristic of ingested polyphenols.

Quercetin has been shown to have effects of antiviral, anti-cancer and anti-inflammatory and to reduce blood pressure in hypertensive and obese subjects in whom low-density lipoprotein cholesterol levels were also reduced. Also, quercetin is monoamine-oxidase inhibitor.

Effect of Various Flavonoids on Bone Tissues

Quercetin has been shown to have effects on bone tissues *in vitro*. The effect of various polyphenols on calcium content and alkaline phosphatase activity in the femoral-diaphyseal and -metaphyseal tissues of young rats *in vitro* has been investigated [152]. Bone tissues were cultured for 24 hours in serum-free Dulbecco's modified Eagle's medium containing either vehicle or various polyphenols (10^{-7} - 10^{-4} M). The presence of genistein (10^{-6} - 10^{-4} M) caused a significant increase in calcium content and alkaline phosphatase activity in the femoral-diaphyseal and -metaphyseal tissues [152]. Resveratrol (10^{-4} M) decreased metaphyseal calcium content significantly, and it (10^{-6} - 10^{-4} M) had a significant inhibitory effect on the diaphyseal enzyme activity [152]. Epigallocatechin gallate (EGCg; 10^{-4} M) significantly inhibited alkaline phosphatase activity in the diaphyseal and metaphyseal tissues [152]. EGCg (10^{-7} - 10^{-4} M) had no effect on bone calcium content [152]. Meanwhile, glycitein, quercetin, or catechin in the range of 10^{-7} to 10^{-4} M did not have an effect on calcium content and alkaline phosphatase activity in the femoral-diaphyseal and -metaphyseal tissues [152]. These findings suggest that, among various flavonoid factors, an isoflavone genistein has a unique anabolic effect on bone calcification in bone tissues *in vitro*. The effect of genistein on bone has been detailed in Chapter 3.

Meanwhile, the effect of various flavonoids, which are present in food and plants, on bone calcium content and osteoclastogenesis has been shown *in vitro* [303]. Rat femoral-diaphyseal (cortical bone) and -metaphyseal (trabecular bone) tissues were cultured for 48 hours in Dulbecco's modified Eagle's medium (high glucose) supplemented with antibiotics and bovine serum albumin. Among quercetin, myricetin, kaempferol, isorhamnetin, curcumin, hesperidin, or astaxanthin in the range of 10^{-7}-10^{-5} M, culture with quercetin (10^{-6} or 10^{-5} M) caused a significant increase in the diaphyseal calcium content [303]. Such effect was not seen in other compounds [303].

Mouse bone marrow cells were cultured for 7 days in the presence of parathyroid hormone (PTH; 10^{-7} M), a bone-resorbing factor, *in vitro* [303]. Culture with PTH caused a significant increase in osteoclast-like cell formation. This increase was significantly suppressed in the presence of quercetin, myricetin, kaempferol, isorhamnetin, or curcumin in the range of 10^{-8} -10^{-6} M [303]. Such an effect was not seen in case of hesperidin or astaxanthin [303]. In addition, culture with PTH (10^{-7} M) caused a significant decrease in the diaphyseal calcium content. This decrease was completely prevented in the presence of quercetin, myricetin, kaempferal, or isorhamnetin with the concentration of 10^{-6} M [303]. This study demonstrates that various flavonoids have an inhibitory effect on osteoclastogenesis and bone resorption rather than bone formation *in vitro*. Among various flavonoids, quercetin has been found to have a stimulatory effect on bone formation and an inhibitory effect on bone resorption *in vitro*.

It has been hypothesized that flavonoids increase bone mass and prevent osteoporosis. However, little is known about the *in vitro* effects of flavonoids on osteoclast activities. The effects of quercetin, one of the most commonly occurring flavonoids, on osteoclast differentiation, which is a critical determinant step of *in vivo* bone resorption have been examined [304]. Two *in vitro* models of osteoclast differentiation were used in this study: a murine one, involving the culture of RAW 264.7 cells in the presence of receptor activator of NF kappa B ligand (RANKL), and a human model consisting of differentiating peripheral blood monocytic cells (PBMC) isolated from peripheral blood in the presence of RANKL and macrophage-colony stimulating factor (M-CSF). Osteoclastogenesis was assessed with osteoclast-like number, tartrate resistant acid phosphatase (TRAP) activity, and bone resorbing activity. Quercetin (0.1-10 μM) decreased osteoclastogenesis in a dose dependent manner in both models with significant effects observed at low concentrations, from 1 to 5 μM. The IC (50) value was about 1 μM. The analysis of protein-DNA interaction by electrophoretic mobility shift assay (EMSA) performed on RAW cells showed that a pre-treatment with quercetin inhibited RANKL-induced nuclear factor κB (NF-κB) and activator protein 1 (AP-1) activation. NF-κB and AP-1 are transcription factors highly involved in osteoclastic differentiation, and their inhibition could play an important role in the decrease of osteoclastogenesis observed in the presence of quercetin. Such finding demonstrates for the first time that quercetin, a flavonoid characterized by antioxidant activities, is a potent inhibitor of *in vitro* osteoclastic differentiation, via a mechanism involving NF-κB and AP-1.

Quercetin, a Potent Suppressor of NF-κB and Smad Activations in Osteoblasts

Many naturally occurring nutritional factors and chemicals isolated from plants are now under investigation for their medicinal properties. The flavonoid quercetin is one of such agent and has been found to possess potent anti-inflammatory effects [305, 306], due in part to its anti-NF-κB activity [306]. The NF-κB signal transduction pathway is synonymous with inflammation and mediates the effect of multiple inflammatory cytokines including RANKL and TNF-α, two cytokines that have potent effects on the skeleton. Skeletal deterioration is common in inflammatory states including rheumatoid arthritis and periodontitis and in postmenopausal osteoporosis where estrogen deficiency leads to upregulation in TNF-α and RANKL [3].

At the cellular level, osteoclasts, that degrade (resorb) bone, are derived from precursors of the monocytic lineage that differentiation into mature osteoclasts under the influence of the key osteoclastogenic cytokine RANKL. TNF-α synergizes with RANKL at the level of signal transduction to amplify its osteoclastogenic activity. NF-κB is a major signal transduction pathway for both cytokines and consequently NF-κB activation is necessary to generate osteoclasts and to regulate their functional activity [307-311].

As described above, some studies have reported that quercetin antagonizes bone resorption in femoral organ cultures [303] and in osteoclast differentiation and/or activation assays *in vitro* [312, 313] by a mechanism that involves suppression of NF-κB and AP-1 [314]. Interestingly, a quercetin-like varient, quercetin-6-C-beta-D-glucopyranoside, which was isolated from Ulmus wallichiana planchon, has been demonstrated to possess enhanced anti-osteoclastogenic activity and to mitigate ovariectomy-induced bone loss in rats [315].

In contrast to osteoclasts, osteoblasts that build and regenerate bone are potently inhibited by TNF-α [284] and it has been demonstrated that mice deficient in TNF-α or its type I receptor achieve a significantly higher bone mineral density as a consequence of elevated bone formation *in vivo* [290]. It has been further demonstrated that pharmacological antagonists of NF-κB activation promote osteoblast differentiation and mineralization *in vitro* [292, 293]. Other studies ratified *in vivo* by a report of time- and stage-specific inhibition of NF-κB activation in differentiated osteoblasts leading to increased trabecular bone mass and bone mineral density [316]. Additional studies have reported increased bone formation and amelioration of osteopenia in ovariectomized mice treated with pharmacological NF-κB inhibitors [317]. Also, in consistent with these data, TNF-α antagonists have been shown to promote bone regeneration in a fracture repair model [318].

However, the action of quercetin on osteoblasts and bone formation is contentious. Quercetin has been reported to inhibit the proliferation, differentiation and mineralization of osteoblasts *in vitro* [319], and to promote TNF-α-induced inhibition [320, 321]. Other studies report an increase in alkaline phosphatase activity (an early osteoblast differentiation marker) in human MG-63 osteoblast cells [322] and stimulatory effects on bone formation in rat organ cultures *ex vivo* [303].

The author *et al.* compared the effects of quercetin on osteoclastogenesis and on osteoblast differentiation [323]. The effect of quercetin on *in vitro* osteoblast differentiation and activity was assessed by treating MC3T3 cells with quercetin at (0.1, 1, 10, or 50 μM) in mineralizing medium for 21 days followed by Alizarin Red-S staining for calcium deposition. The data showed that between 0.1 and 10 μM quercetin had no effect on mineralization, but at 50 μM had a suppressive activity on the differentiation of MC3T3 cells into mineralizing osteoblasts [323].

TGF-β and BMP-2 are early and late osteoblast commitment and differentiation factors respectively and both signal in large measure though the Smad pathway, albeit though different R-Smads. The effect of quercetin on BMP-2- and TGF-β-induced Smad activation was assessed in MC3T3 cells transfected with a Smad-luciferase reporter [323]. Surprisingly, quercetin alone elicited a direct potent dose responsive (0.1 to 25 μM) suppression of both BMP-2- and TGF-β-induced Smad activation.

The effect of quercetin has also been examined in osteoclast formation using the RAW264.7 cell line, which differentiates into mature multinucleated osteoclasts when treated with RANKL [323]. Quercetin potently and dose-dependently inhibited RANKL-induced osteoclastogenesis in the range (0.1, 1, 10, and 25 μM) [323]. Consistent with the osteoclastogenesis assays quercetin antagonized RANKL-induced NF-κB activation in the dose range (0.1, 1, 10, and 50 μM) in preosteoclastic RAW264.7 cells [323].

Quercetin has been reported to suppress osteoclastogenesis *in vitro* and prevent bone loss in ovariectomized mice *in vivo*. By contrast, the effect of quercetin on osteoblasts, the cells responsible for bone formation, is contradictory with conflicting reports of inhibition as well as stimulation. Given previous reports that NF-κB antagonists promote osteoblast differentiation and activity, the author *et al.* compared the effects of quercetin on osteoclast and osteoblast differentiation and on NF-κB signal transduction *in vitro*. As expected, quercetin potently suppressed osteoclastogenesis and NF-κB activation induced by RANKL in osteoclast precursors [323]. However, the same doses of quercetin had no effect on osteoblast mineralization, and failed to significantly alleviate the inhibitory effect of NF-κB-induced by TNF-α, even though quercetin potently suppressed NF-κB activation in these cells [323]. This apparent contradiction was explained by the fact that addition to its anti-NF-κB activity; quercetin also potently antagonized both TGF-β and BMP-2-induced Smad activation in osteoblast precursors. Taken together our data suggest that multiple competing actions of quercetin mediate both stimulatory and inhibitory actions on osteoblasts with the final physiological effect likely a function of the net balance between these stimulatory and inhibitory effects.

The author *et al.* have shown that TNF-α suppresses osteoblast differentiation, in part, by antagonizing Smad activation by BMP-2 and TGF-β. Quercetin failed to alleviate the suppressive action of TNF-α on BMP-2-induced, or TGF-β-induced Smad-activation [323]. In fact, quercetin significantly amplified the inhibitory effect of TNF-α on Smad activation induced by both cytokines [323].

The effect of quercetin on osteoblast differentiation is less clear cut with both suppression and stimulation being report [319-322]. While our data did indeed validate a potent suppressive effect of quercetin on TNF-α-induced NF-κB activation, surprisingly this did not translate into a strong bone anabolic effect. Instead quercetin displayed very weak anabolic activity at low dose and even suppressive activity at high dose, although general toxicity was not observed [323].

One mechanism by which TNF-α suppresses osteoblastogenesis is by antagonizing the activation of Smad signal transduction by TGF-β and BMP-2, early commitment [324] and late differentiation [325] factors respectively. Although unexpected, our data are consistent with a previous report in which quercetin inhibited Smad activation in keloid-derived fibroblasts [326].

Taken together our data suggest the existence of complex competing actions of quercetin on osteoblast signal transduction pathways. Ultimately, the net effect of quercetin on osteoblasts *in vitro* and *in vivo* may be dose and context dependent with the prevailing concentrations of competing cytokines and growth factors in the bone marrow microenvironment determining whether the final effect is stimulatory or inhibitory to bone formation.

The specific mechanisms by which quercetin is able to modulate both NF-κB and Smad, and potential other signaling systems remains to be determined, and may ultimately facilitate the rational design of antagonists possessing either NF-κB or Smad inhibitory actions for use as anti-inflammatory pharmaceuticals to ameliorate bone loss and other diseases associated with inflammation.

Role of Dietary Quercetin in Osteoporosis Treatment

Flavonoids are micronutrients widely present in food of plant origin. They have been attributed pharmacological properties such as anticancer and prevention of age-related pathologies. Quercetin is a major dietary flavonoid found in onions and other vegetables, and potentially has beneficial effects on disease prevention.

The effects of dietary quercetin on bone loss and uterine weight loss by ovariectomy *in vivo* have been shown [327]. Female mice were ovariectomized (OVX) and were randomly allocated to 3 groups: a control diet or a diet with 0.25% (LQ) or 2.5% quercetin (HQ). After 4 weeks, dietary quercetin had no effects on uterine weight in OVX mice, but bone mineral density of the lumbar spine L4 and femur measured by peripheral quantitative computed tomography (pQCT) was higher in both the sham and the HQ groups than in the OVX group. Histomorphometric analysis showed that the HQ group restored bone volume (BV/TV) completely in distal femoral cancellous bone, but did not reduce the osteoclast surface area and osteoclast number when compared with the OVX group [327].

In *in-vitro* experiments using mouse monocyte/macrophage cell line RAW264.7 cells, however, quercetin and their conjugate, quercetin-3-O-beta-D: -glucuronide dose-dependently inhibited the receptor activator of RANKL-induced osteoclast differentiation, and the RANKL-stimulated expression of osteoclast related genes was also inhibited by quercetin [327]. The luciferase reporter assay showed that quercetin did not appear to have estrogenic activity through estrogen receptors [327]. These results suggest that dietary quercetin inhibits bone loss without effect on the uterus in OVX mice and does not act as a potent inhibitor of osteoclastogenesis or as a selective estrogen receptor modulator *in vivo* [327].

The effects of standardized and concentrated extract of Ginkgo biloba, Egb 761, were studied on estrogen deficiency-induced bone loss in ovariectomized (OVX) rats rendered osteopenic [328]. Upon osteopenia development, Egb 761 was administered at a dose of 100 mg/kg/day by oral gavage to OVX rats whereas control group received vehicle. Following 5 weeks of treatment, the OVX + Egb 761 group (n=12) of rats exhibited significantly higher whole body bone mineral density (BMD) and lower bone turnover markers (serum alkaline phosphatase and osteocalcin) than OVX rats that were given vehicle (n=12) [328]. BMD levels in excised bones were also found to be higher in both trabecular (most robustly in lumbar vertebrae) and cortical bones of OVX + Egb 761 compared with OVX+vehicle group [328]. Egb 761 did not exhibit estrogen agonistic activity at the uterine level [328]. Microcomputed tomography demonstrated that OVX + Egb 761 group had better bone microarchitectural parameters compared with OVX + vehicle group [328]. Moreover, OVX – Egb 761 group had higher femoral mRNA levels of osterix, type I collagen and osteocalcin compared with OVX+vehicle group [328]. Determination of levels of three flavonoids of Egb

761, that are known to have bone conserving property, in serum and bone marrow suggests that kaempferol and quercetin, and not rutin, likely mediate the beneficial actions observed with Egb 761 treatment [328]. These observations show for the first time that oral administration of Egb 761 restores bone mass in aged OVX rats.

6-C-β-D-glucopyranosyl-(2S,3S)-(+)-3',4',5,7-tetrahydroxyflavanol (GTDF), a novel flavonol-C-glucoside isolated from the plant extracts, has a nonestrogenic bone-sparing effect on OVX rats [329]. The effects of GTDF on osteoblast function and its mode of action and *in vivo* osteogenic effect have been examined [329]. GTDF stimulated osteoblast proliferation, survival, and differentiation but had no effect on osteoclastic or adipocytic differentiation [329]. In cultured osteoblasts, GTDF transactivated the aryl hydrocarbon receptor (AhR) [329]. Activation of AhR mediated the stimulatory effect of GTDF on osteoblast proliferation and differentiation [329]. Furthermore, GTDF stimulated cAMP production, which mediated osteogenic gene expression. GTDF treatments given to 1- to 2-day-old rats or adult rats increased the mRNA levels of AhR target genes in calvaria or bone marrow stromal cells [329]. In growing female rats, GTDF promoted parameters of peak bone accrual in the appendicular skeleton, including increased longitudinal growth, bone mineral density, bone-formation rate (BFR), cortical deposition, and bone strength [329]. GTDF promoted the process of providing newly generated bone to fill drill holes in the femurs of both estrogen-sufficient and -deficient rats [329]. In osteopenic OVX rats, GTDF increased BFR and significantly restored trabecular bone compared with the ovaries-intact group [329]. Together these data suggest that GTDF stimulates osteoblast growth and differentiation via the AhR and promotes modeling-directed bone accrual, accelerates bone healing after injury, and exerts anabolic effects on osteopenic rats likely by a direct stimulatory effect on osteoprogenitors [329].

Diabetic osteopenia can result in an increased incidence of bone fracture and a delay in fracture healing. Quercetin, one of the most widely distributed flavonoids in plants, possesses antioxidant property and beneficial effect on osteoporosis in ovariectomized mice. All these properties make quercetin a potential candidate for controlling the development of diabetic osteopenia [330]. The putative beneficial effect of quercetin on diabetic osteopenia in rats has been examined [330]. Diabetes mellitus was induced by streptozotocin. The diabetic rats received daily oral administration of quercetin (5, 30, and 50 mg/kg body weight) for 8 weeks, which was started at 4 weeks after streptozotocin injection [330]. Quercetin at 5 mg/kg showed little effect on diabetic osteopenia, while quercetin at 30 and 50 mg/kg could increase the decreased serum osteocalcin, serum alkaline phosphatase activity, and urinary deoxypyridinoline in diabetic rats [330]. In addition, quercetin (30 and 50 mg/kg) could partially reverse the decreased biomechanical quality and the impaired micro-architecture of the femurs in diabetic rats [330]. Histomorphometric analysis showed that both decreased bone formation and resorption were observed in diabetic rats, which was partially restored by quercetin (30 and 50mg/kg) [330]. Further investigations showed that quercetin significantly lowered the oxidative DNA damage level, up-regulated the total serum antioxidant capability and the activity of serum antioxidants in diabetic rats [330]. All those findings indicate the beneficial effect of quercetin on diabetic osteopenia in rats, and raise the possibility of developing quercetin as potential drugs or an ingredient in diet for controlling diabetic osteopenia [330].

Other experiment has been conducted to observe the effects of rutin (quercetin-3-O-glucose rhamnose) on bone metabolism in ovariectomized (OVX) rats [331]. Thirty 3-month-old Wistar rats were used. Twenty were OVX while the 10 controls were sham-operated (SH). Among the 20 OVX, for 90 days after surgery 10 were fed the same synthetic diet as the SH or OVX ones, but 0. 25% rutin (OVX + R) was added. At necropsy, the decrease in uterine weight was not different in OVX and OVX + R rats [331]. OVX also induced a significant decrease in both total and distal metaphyseal femoral mineral density, which was prevented by rutin consumption [331]. Moreover, femoral failure load, which was not different in OVX and SH rats, was even higher in OVX + R rats than in OVX or SH rats [331]. In the same way, on day 90, both urinary deoxypyridinoline (DPD) excretion (a marker for bone resorption) and calciuria were higher in OVX rats than in OVX + R or SH rats [331]. Simultaneously, plasma osteocalcin (OC) concentration (a marker for osteoblastic activity) was higher in OVX + R rats than in SH rats [331]. High-performance liquid chromatography profiles of plasma samples from OVX + R rats revealed that mean plasma concentration of active metabolites (quercetin and isorhamnetin) from rutin was 9.46+/-1 μM, whereas it was undetectable in SH and OVX rats [331]. These findings indicate that rutin (and/or its metabolites), which appeared devoid of any uterotrophic activity, inhibits ovariectomy-induced trabecular bone loss in rats, both by slowing down resorption and increasing osteoblastic activity [331].

Conclusion

Flavonoid, a kind of polyphenol, possesses a fundmental chemical structure of flavone and displays yellow pigments, including flavone, isoflavon, flavonol, flavonon and quercetin, which are found in fruits, vegetables, leaves and grains. Flavonoid has a strong anti-oxidant effect. In recent years, flavonoid has been shown to have an effect on bone. Quercetin, a flavonol, is a plant-derived flavonoid. It is used as an ingredient in supplements, beverages or foods. Quercetin has been shown to have a stimulatory effect on osteoblastic bone formation and a suppressive effect on osteoclastic bone resorption. Quercetin suppresses NF-κB activation, which is mediated through TNF-α and RANKL in osteoblastogenesis and osteoclastogenesis. Oral administration of quercetin has been shown to have preventive and treatment effects on estrogen deficiency-induced bone loss in ovariectomized animals, a model of menopausal osteoporosis. Supplemental intake of dietary quercetin may have a role in the treatment of osteoporosis.

Chapter 9

Role of Ginger Factor Curcumin in Osteoporosis Treatment

Curcumin is the principal curcuminoid of the popular Indian spice turmeric, which is a member of the ginger family (*Zingiberaceae*). Turmeric's other two curcuminoids are desmethoxycurcumin and bis-desmethoxycurcumin. The curcuminoids are natural phenols that are responsible for the yellow color of turmeric. Curcumin can exist in several tautomeric forms, including a 1, 3-diketo form and two equivalent enol forms. The enol form is more energetically stable in the solid phase and in solution. Curcumin can be used for boron quantification in the curcumin method. It reacts with boric acid to form a red-colored compound, rosocyanine.

The biosynthetic route of curcumin has proven to be very difficult for researchers to determine. In 1973, Roughly and Whiting proposed mechanism for curcumin biosynthesis. The mechanism involved two cinnamate units being coupled together by malonyl-CoA. The mechanism uses cinnamic acid as their starting point, which is derived from the amino acid phenylalanine. This is noteworthy because plant biosyntheses employing cinnamic acid as a starting point are rare compared to the more common use of *p*-coumaric acid. Only a few identified compounds, such as anigorufone and pinosylvin, use cinnamic acid as their start molecule.

Biological Effects of Curcumin

Curcumin may be useful for the prevention and treatment of several diseases [332, 333]. The effectiveness of curcumin has neither been confirmed in sufficient preliminary research, and it has been not demonstrated in randomized, placebo-controlled, and double-blind clinical trials. In one preliminary study, a daily dose of 2 grams of curcumin extract was found to provide pain relief that was equivalent to ibuprofen for the relief of pain associated with osteoarthritis of the knee. A survey of the literature shows a number of other potential uses and that daily doses over a 3-month period of up to 12 grams proved safe. Some commercial capsules of curcumin contain piperine, a compound found in pepper which aids absorption of curcumin into the blood stream. However, as curcuma is known to inhibit blood clotting, it should be avoided for a two-week period prior to major surgery and not used in conjunction with blood thinners. Curcumin may also affect gallstone formation.

Several preliminary research studies have identified curcumin with potential biological effects. *In vitro* and animal studies have suggested potential biological effects associated with curcumin. At present, these effects have not been confirmed in humans. As of 2008, clinical trials in humans were underway, studying the effect of curcumin on various diseases, including multiple myeloma, pancreatic cancer, myelodysplastic syndromes, colon cancer, psoriasis, and Alzheimer's disease. In both *in vitro* and animal studies, curcumin has shown antitumor, antioxidant, antiarthritic, antiamyloid, anti-ischemic, and anti-inflammatory properties. Anti-inflammatory properties may be due to inhibition of eicosanoid biosynthesis.

The effect of curcumin on β-amyloid plaque build up, a possible major cause for Alzheimer's disease has been studied in mice. According to theory, curcumin may provide anti-inflammatory effects in a neuro-inflammatory cascade in plaque pathogenesis. The study demonstrated that both low and high doses of curcumin reduced β-amyloid plaque buildup, an effect that may be similar to that of aspirin which suppressed development of β-amyloid plaque buildup in preliminary research.

The potential anticancer effects of curcumin have been the subject of several preliminary studies. Its potential anticancer effects may stem from an ability to induce apoptosis in cancer cells without cytotoxic effects on healthy cells. Curcumin may interfere with activity of the transcription factor NF-κB, which has been linked to a number of inflammatory diseases such as cancer.

In Phase I clinical trials, dietary curcumin was shown to exhibit poor bioavailability (i.e., low levels in plasma and tissues). Potential factors that limit the bioavailability of curcumin include poor absorption, rapid metabolism, and rapid systemic elimination. Numerous approaches to increasing curcumin bioavailability have been explored, including the use of adjuvants like piperine. The bioavailability of curcumin ingested in foods may be increased as a result of cooking or dissolution in oil.

Curcumin, like many antioxidants, can be a "double-edged sword" where, in the test tube, carcinogenic and pro-oxidant effects may be seen in addition to anticancer and antioxidant effects. *In vitro* and *in vivo* studies suggest that curcumin can have carcinogenic effects.

Effect of Curcumin on Bone Homeostasis

Bone homeostasis is maintained through a delicate balance between osteoblastic bone formation and osteoclastic bone resorption. Numerous pathological processes have the capacity to disrupt this equilibrium leading to conditions where the rate of bone resorption outpaces the rate of bone formation leading to osteoporosis that is induced with decrease in bone mass. Postmenopausal osteoporosis, a consequence of ovarian hormone deficiency, is the archetypal osteoporotic condition in women after menopause and leads to bone destruction though complex and diverse metabolic and biochemical changes [1-3]. The most dramatic expression of osteoporosis is represented by fractures of the proximal femur for which the number increases as the population ages. Pharmacologic and functional food factors may have the potential effect to delay degenerative bone disorders such as osteoporosis. Curcumin has been found to suppress osteoclastogenesis in bone marrow cell culture *in vitro* [303], suggesting a role of curcumin in the prevention and treatment in osteoporosis.

Effect of Curcumin in Osteoblastgenesis

Curcumin is a phenolic natural product isolated from the rhizome of Curcuma longa (turmeric) and has effects on bone health and fat formation. The bone marrow mesenchymal stem cells are multipotent cells capable of differentiating into osteoblasts and adipocytes. Osteoblast differentiation of bone marrow mesenchymal stem cells can be a result of upregulation of heme oxygenase (HO)-1 expression. Curcumin can potently induce HO-1 expression. The study describes the effects of curcumin on differentiation of rat bone marrow mesenchymal stem cells into osteoblasts and adipocytes [332]. Rat bone marrow mesenchymal stem cells were isolated and treated with or without curcumin. Osteoblast differentiation was confirmed and determined by alkaline phosphatase (ALP) activity, mineralized nodule formation, the expression of Runx2 (runt-related transcription factor 2) and osteocalcin. Adipocyte differentiation was determined by Oil red O staining and the expression of peroxisome proliferator-activated receptor-γ 2 (PPARγ2) and CCAAT/enhancer-binding protein (C/EBP) α. Curcumin increased ALP activity and osteoblast-specific mRNA expression of Runx2 and osteocalcin when rat bone marrow mesenchymal stem cells were cultured in osteogenic medium [332]. In contrast, curcumin decreased adipocyte differentiation and inhibited adipocyte-specific mRNA expression of PPARγ2 and C/EBPα when rMSCs were cultured in adipogenic medium [332]. HO-1 expression was increased during osteogenic differentiation of rat bone marrow mesenchymal stem cells. These findings demonstrate that curcumin can promote osteogenic differentiation of bone marrow mesenchymal stem cells and inhibit adipocyte formation. The effect of curcumin on osteogenic differentiation of bone marrow mesenchymal stem cells is correlated with HO-1 expression.

Curcumin (diferuloylmethane) is found in the rhizomes of the turmeric plant (Curcuma longa L.) and has been used for centuries as a dietary spice and as a traditional Indian medicine used to treat different conditions [333]. At the cellular level, curcumin modulates important molecular targets: transcription factors, enzymes, cell cycle proteins, cytokines, receptors and cell surface adhesion molecules [333]. Because many of the curcumin targets mentioned above participate in the regulation of bone remodeling, curcumin may affect the skeletal system. Nitric oxide (NO) is a gaseous molecule generated from L-arginine during the catalization of nitric oxide synthase (NOS), and it plays crucial roles in catalization and in the nervous, cardiovascular and immune systems [333]. Human osteoblasts have been shown to express NOS isoforms, and the exact mechanism(s) by which NO regulates bone formation remain unclear. Curcumin has been widely described to inhibit inducible NO synthase expression and NO production, at least in part via direct interference in NF-κB activation [333]. It has been observed that curcumin abrogated inducible NOS expression and decreased NO levels, inhibiting also cell prolifieration after exposure of human osteoblast-like cells (MG-63) [333]. This effect was prevented by the NO donor sodium nitroprusside [333]. Under osteogenic conditions, curcumin also decreased the level of mineralization [333], although these results indicate that NO plays a role in the osteoblastic profile of MG-63 cells [333].

Thus, it has been reported that curcumin has stimulatory or suppressive effects on osteoblastogenesis in osteblastic cells *in vitro.*

Effect of Curcumin in Osteoclastogenesis

Curcumin is a potent inhibitor of the transcriptional factors activator protein-1 (AP-1) and nuclear factor-kappaB (NF-κB). Since transcriptional factors may play a functional role in the survival of osteoclasts, the effect of curcumin on osteoclast apoptosis has been examined [334]. It has been observed that curcumin is a potent stimulator of this process in rabbit osteoclasts, as evidenced by morphological changes in nuclei and DNA fragmentation as criteria of apoptosis [334]. The curcumin stimulation of the osteoclast apoptosis was dose-and treatment time-dependent [334]. In addition, curcumin dramatically inhibited osteoclastic bone resorption, supporting the view that curcumin is a potent stimulator of osteoclast apoptosis [334].

Numerous studies have indicated that inflammatory cytokines play a major role in osteoclastogenesis, leading to the bone resorption that is frequently associated with cancers and other diseases. Gene deletion studies have shown that receptor activator of NF-kappaB ligand (RANKL) is one of the critical mediators of osteoclastogenesis. It has been examined whether curcumin (diferuloylmethane), a pigment derived from turmeric, has suppressive effects on RANKL signaling and osteoclastogenesis in RAW 264.7 cells, a murine monocytic cell line [335]. Treatment of these cells with RANKL activated NF-κB, and preexposure of the cells to curcumin completely suppressed RANKL-induced NF-κB activation [335]. Curcumin inhibited the pathway leading from activation of IκBα kinase and IκBα phosphorylation to IκBα degradation [335]. RANKL induced osteoclastogenesis in these monocytic cells, and curcumin inhibited both RANKL- and TNF-α-induced osteoclastogenesis and pit formation [335]. Curcumin suppressed osteoclastogenesis maximally when added together with RANKL and minimally when it was added 2 days after RANKL [335]. Whether curcumin inhibits RANKL-induced osteoclastogenesis through suppression of NF-κB was also confirmed independently, as RANKL failed to activate NF-κB in cells stably transfected with a dominant-negative form of IκBα and concurrently failed to induce osteoclastogenesis [335]. Thus, overall these findings indicate that RANKL induces osteoclastogenesis through the activation of NF-κB, and treatment with curcumin inhibits both the NF-κB activation and osteoclastogenesis induced by RANKL.

Effect of Novel Curcumin Analogues in Bone Homeostasis

Pharmacologic and functional food factors may have the potential effect to delay degenerative bone disorders such as osteoporosis. Compound, which is newly synthesized from functional food factors, may have potential effects in the prevention and treatment of osteoporosis, suggesting the usefulness as a pharmacologic tool.

Newly curcumin analogues including EF31, MCNN 909, and UBS109 from curcumin, a functional food factor have been synthesized [336-338]. These chemical structures are shown in Figure 21.

EF31 has been found to have an inhibitory effect on NF-κB signaling in cancer cells [337]. However, the action of these curcumin analogues on bone cells has not been reported so far. The author *et al.* found that UBS109 has potential effects on the stimulation of osteoblastogenesis and the suppression of osteoclastogenesis *in vitro*, suggesting a useful tool as new compound in the prevention and treatment of osteolysis and osteopolosis.

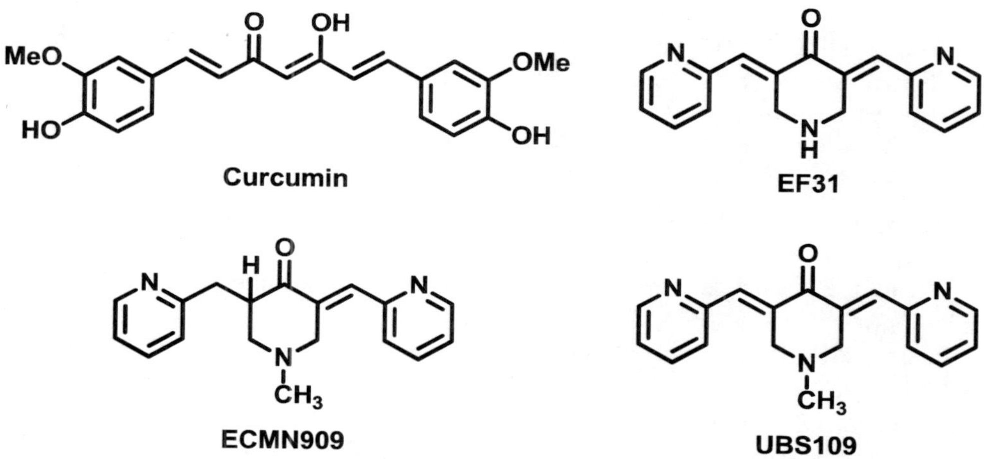

Figure 21. Structure of curcumin and its related compounds. The molecular weigh of cucumin, EF31, MCNN909, and UBS109 is 368.38, 277.32, 293.36, and 291.35, respectively.

Effect of Curcumin Analogues in Osteoblastogenesis

The direct effect of curcumin analogues on bone formation and mineralization has been examined. To address this issue the author *et al.* investigated the action of curcumin analogues (curcumin, EF31, ECMN909 and UBS109) on osteoblast differentiation and mineralization *in vitro*. MC3T3 preosteoblastic cells were differentiated into mineralizing osteoblasts *in vitro* in the presence or absence of curcumin analogues (10 or 100 nM) in mineralizing medium for 21 days and stained for calcium deposition with Alizarin Red-S [339]. UBS109 was found to potently enhance mineralization in both MC3T3 cells [339]. UBS109 did not appear to mediate direct toxic effects on the cultures as cells proliferated robustly over the culture period, and were still alive and visibly attached to the plate at the end of the experiment.

BMPs such as BMP-2 are anabolic agents that signal through the Smad signaling pathway [12]. The author *et al.* thus examined the effect of curcumin analogs on basal and BMP-2-induced Smad activation using a Smad 4-luciferase reporter responsive to all Smad species [339]. Interestingly, UBS109 had a direct effect on basal Smad activation [339]. It potently and significantly enhanced Smad activation induced by BMP-2 or TGF-β1 [339]. However, curcumin, EF31, and MCNN909 did not have an effect on basal Smad and BMP-2-

induced Smad activation [339]. Curcumin analogues did not have the luciferase activity in empty vector control (pGL3-Basic).

Thus, a new action of curcumin analogue UBS109, an *in vitro* capacity to stimulate osteoblastic differentiation and mineralization has been demonstrated. UBS 109 was potently effective in promoting osteoblast mineralization with the dose-dependency (10 and 100 nM) as compared with that of other curcumin analogues (curcumin, EF31, and ECMN909) [339]. BMP2- or TGF-β1-induced Smad signaling respectively plays an important role in the early commitment and differentiation of osteoblasts [12]. UBS109 stimulated both basal Smad activity and BMP-induced Smad activation with the dose-dependency (10 - 500 nM), although such an effect was not seen with other curcumin analogues [339]. UBS109 also enhanced TGF-β-induced Smad activation [339]. UBS109-induced Smad activation may be an important to stimulate osteoblastic differentiation and mineralization [339], suggesting a molecular mechanism.

NF-κB activation is potently inhibitory to osteoblast differentiation, and TNF-α-induced NF-κB activation leads to Smad suppression in MC3T3 osteoblast precursors [13]. We next investigated whether UBS109 is able to prevent TNF-α-induced Smad suppression in MC3T3 osteoblast precursors [339]. UBS109 significantly prevented TNF-α-induced Smad suppression [339]. Such an effect was not seen in case of curcumin, EF31, and MCNN 909 [339].

Because NF-κB activation is potently inhibitory to osteoblast differentiation [13], we next investigated whether curcumin analogue is able to suppress basal and/or intensify TNF-α-induced NF-κB activation in MC3T3 osteoblast precursors [339]. MC3T3 cells were transiently transfected with an NF-κB luciferase reporter and luciferase activity was quantitated in the presence or absence of curcumin analogue. Curcumin did not have an effect on basal NF-κB activity and TNF-α-induced increase in NF-κB activity [339]. UBS109 (1 and 10 μM) significantly suppressed basal NF-κB activity and TNF-α-induced NF-κB activity [339]. Such an effect was also seen at 10 μM with higher concentration of EF31 or ECMN 909 [339].

NF-κB signaling has been shown to downregulate osteoblast differentiation [290]. One major mechanism appears to involve the intersection of NF-κB with the Smad signaling pathway [290]. NF-κB signaling in osteoblasts intersects with and disrupts Smad signaling by promoting production of Smad7, an inhibitor of TGF-β- and BMP-induced R-Smad activation [291]. TNF-α further antagonizes BMP signaling by upregulating Smad ubiquitination regulatory factor 1 (Smurf1), promoting proteasomal degradation of bone morphogenetic signaling proteins [340]. Multiple suppressors of NF-κB activation are capable of rescuing the inhibitory effect of TNF-α on BMP-2 and/or TGF-β1-induced Smad activation [340, 341]. UBS109 was found to prevent TNF-α-induced Smad suppression that is partly related to the mechanism by which UBS109 stimulates osteoblastic differentiation and mineralization [339].

EF 31 and ECMN909 with 10 μM was found to suppress in basal NF-κB activity and TNF-α-induced NF-κB activation [339]. The suppressive effect of UBS 109 on NF-κB activation was seen at the dose of 1 and 10 μM [339]. The effect of UBS109 was potently as compared with that of other compounds [339]. The reversible effect of UBS 109 on TNF-α-induced Smad suppression was revealed with the dose of over 10 nM [339]. UBS 109 may have a potential-direct effect on Smad activation rather than NF-κB suppression. It cannot exclude, however, that the stimulatory effect of UBS109 on osteoblastic mineralization may be partly related to the suppressive effect of the compound on TNF-α-induced NF-κB activation.

Effect of Curcumin Analogues in Osteoclastogenesis

To examine the effect of curcumin analogues on osteoclast formation, RAW264.7 osteoclast precursors were differentiated into mature osteoclasts by stimulation with RANKL in the presence or absence of curcumin analogue with the dose 50 and 100 nM. Curcumin analogues with 100 nM did not have a toxic to the precursors suppressing their proliferation over 7 days of culture [339]. Curcumin was not significantly reduced osteoclast formation in the dose of 100 nM [339]. EF31 of 100 nM, ECMN909 of 50 and 100 nM, and UBS109 with the dose 50 to 100 nM significantly suppressed osteoclast formation [339].

The NF-κB signal transduction pathway is essential for the generation of osteoclasts [14, 15]. The effect of curcumin analogues on NF-κB activation by RANKL in osteoclast precursors was examined. RAW 264.7 cells were transfected with an NF-κB reporter and stimulated with RANKL to induce NF-κB activity, in the presence or absence of curcumin analogues [339]. Basal and RANKL-induced increase in NF-κB activity was not significantly blunted in the presence of curcumin (50 and 100 nM) [339]. Basal activity was suppressed with EF31 (100 nM) and ECMN909 (100 nM), and it was decreased with UBS109 (500 nM) [339]. RANKL-induced increase in NF-κB activity was significantly suppressed in the presence of EF31 (100 nM), ECMN 909 (50 and 100 nM) or UBS 109 (50 and 100 nM) [339]. Thus, ECMN909 and UBS 109 had a potent-suppressive effect on RANKL-induced NF-κB activation in osteoclast precursor cells.

Curcumin has been reported to inhibit osteoclastogenesis by decreasing RANKL signaling in bone marrow stromal cells [342]. Curcumin analogues (EF 31, ECMN909 and UBS109) with dose-dependency (50-500 nM), which did not have cell toxicity, were found to have a suppressive effect on osteoclastogenesis, although the effect of curcumin was seen with only higher dose (500 nM) [339]. RANKL, the key osteoclastogenic cytokine, is central to formation of osteoclasts, the cells that resorb bone, through NF-κB signaling [14, 15]. Curcumin analogues with the dose-dependency suppressed RANKL-induced NF-κB activation in osteoclast precursor cells [339]. ECMN909 and UBS109 (50 and100 nM) potently suppressed RANKL-induced NF-κB activation in osteoclast precursor cells as compared with that of curcumin and EF31 [339]. This finding coincided with the observation of their suppressive effect of osteoclastogenesis, suggesting the mechanism by which ECMN909 and UBS109 suppress osteoclastogenesis [339].

Of various curcumin analogues tested, UBS109 was found to have potential stimulatory effects on osteoblastogenesis and suppressive effects on osteoclastogenesis *in vitro* through Smad activation and NF-κB inhibition, indicating a relationship with chemical structure and bone cell effects. Culture with UBS109 may stimulate the nuclear translocation of Smad4 in osteoblastic cells and may suppress the nuclear translocation of p65 and increase cytoplasma IκB in preosteoclasts. The molecular mechanism by which UBS 109 stimulates Smad signaling and suppresses NF-κB activation remains to be elucidated.

In conclusion, it has been demonstrated that the novel curcumin analogue UBS109 possesses potent Smad and anti-NF-κB activity and may have promise for development into an antiosteoporotic agent capable of promoting new bone formation while simultaneously reducing bone resorption. This compound may be useful as a therapeutic tool in the prevention and treatment of osteolysis with various pathophysiologic states *in vivo*.

Role of Dietary Curcumin in Osteoporosis Treatment

There is increasing interest in the discovery of natural compounds that could favorably affect the skeletal system. Curcumin is a constituent of turmeric, a plant which has been used for centuries as a dietary spice and a traditional Indian medicine. Curcumin has been reported to affect differentiation, activity and the lifespan of osteoblasts and osteoclasts *in vitro*. The effects of curcumin on the skeletal system of rats *in vivo* have been examined [343]. Curcumin (10 mg/kg daily) was orally administered for four weeks to normal (non-ovariectomized) and bilaterally ovariectomized (OVX; estrogen-deficient) 3-month-old female Wistar Cmd: (WI) WU rats [343]. OVX was performed seven days before the start of curcumin administration. Bone mass, mineral and calcium content, macrometric and histomorphometric parameters, as well as the mechanical properties of the bone, were examined [343]. Serum total cholesterol and estradiol levels were also determined. In rats with normal estrogen levels, curcumin decreased serum estradiol level and slightly increased cancellous bone formation, along with decreased mineralization [343]. Estrogen deficiency induced osteoporotic changes in the skeletal system of the ovariectomized control rats [343]. In OVX rats, curcumin decreased body mass gain and serum total cholesterol level, slightly improved some bone histomorphometric parameters impaired by estrogen deficiency, but did not improve bone mineralization or mechanical properties [343]. These observations in *in vivo* study using rats did not support the hypothesis that curcumin, at doses that are readily achievable through dietary intake, could be useful for the prevention or treatment of osteoporosis.

Osteoporosis is a metabolic disease affecting both men and women especially in postmenopausal women. Curcumin possesses many medicinal properties. In this study, thirty two female Sprague-Dawley rats were used to determine the potential effect of curcumin in the prevention of bone loss following ovariectomy [344]. The animals were divided into Sham group, ovariectomised (OVX) control, OVX treated with curcumin 110 mg/kg and ovariectomised treated with Premarin 100 μg/kg [344]. The treatments were given via daily oral gavages for 60 days. The structural parameters such as bone volume, trabecular number, trabecular thickness and trabecular separation were found to be deteriorated in OVX rats compared to Sham group [344]. Moreover, the reduced osteoblast count, the increased osteoclast count and increased eroded surface were found in OVX groups [344]. Treatment with curcumin was able to reverse all these OVX-induced deteriorations [344]. Curcumin treatment was as effective as Premarin in most parameters except the bone volume and eroded surface, which were better than Premarin [344]. The high dose of curcumin treatment was not only able to reduce the osteoclast number but also increase the osteoblast count [344].

Therefore, the potential effect of curcumin can be applied as an alternative to oestrogen for prevention of postmenopausal osteoporosis [344].

Curcumin is a potent inhibitor of the transcription factor activator protein-1 (AP-1) which plays an essential role in osteoclastogenesis [345]. However, the effects of curcumin on bone metabolism have not been clarified *in vivo*. The inhibitory effects of curcumin on the stimulated osteoclastic activity in insulin-dependent diabetes mellitus using rats with streptozotocin-induced diabetes have been reported [345]. A dietary supplement of curcumin reversed the increase in levels of activity and mRNA of tartrate-resistant acid phosphatase (TRAP) and cathepsin K to control values [345]. A histochemical analysis showed that the increase in TRAP-positive cells in the distal femur of the diabetic rats was reduced to the control level by the supplement [345]. These observations suggest that curcumin reduced diabetes-stimulated bone resorptive activity and the number of osteoclasts [345]. When bone marrow cells were cultured with macrophage colony stimulating factor and receptor activator RANKL, the increased activity to form TRAP-positive multinucleated cells and the increased levels of mRNA and protein of c-fos and c-jun in the cultured cells from diabetic rats decreased to control levels in the curcumin-supplemented rats [345]. Similarly, the increased expression of c-fos and c-jun in the distal femur of the diabetic rats was significantly reduced by the supplement [345]. These findings suggested that curcumin suppressed the increased bone resorptive activity through the prevention of osteoclastogenesis associated with inhibition of the expression of c-fos and c-jun in the diabetic rats [345].

Curcumin, an active ingredient of turmeric, is proved to be a potential candidate of controlling inflammation and bone resorption, but few reports are on the periodontitis. It has been evaluated whether the intra-gastric administration of curcumin could inhibit the inflammation and alveolar bone resorption in rats following ligature-induced experimental periodontitis [346]. Male Wistar rats were randomly divided into three groups: no ligature placement and administration of vehicle, ligature placement and administration of vehicle, ligature placement and administration of curcumin [346]. After the animals were sacrificed, their mandibles were collected for morphological, histological and immunohistochemical analysis; their gingival tissues were collected for cytokine measurements. Bone resorption was significantly higher in the experimental periodontitis animals treated with vehicle compared with the curcumin-treated group or the control group [346]. Furthermore, receptor activator of nuclear factor-kapper (κ)B ligand (RANKL), receptor activator of nuclear factor-κB (RANK), osteoprotegerin (OPG), tumor necrosis factor-α (TNF-α) and interleukin-6 (IL-6) expression levels were higher in the experimental periodontitis animals treated with vehicle compared with the curcumin treated group or the control group [346]. Curcumin may decrease alveolar bone loss in the experimental periodontitis rats via suppressing the expression of RANKL/RANK/OPG and its anti-inflammatory properties.

Conclusion

Curcumin is the principal curcuminoid of the popular Indian spice turmeric, which is a member of the ginger family (*Zingiberaceae*). Curcumin may be useful for the prevention and treatment of several diseases. In both *in vitro* and animal studies, curcumin has been shown to have antitumor, antioxidant, antiarthritic, antiamyloid, anti-ischemic, and anti-inflammatory properties. As of 2008, clinical trials in humans were underway, studying the effect of curcumin on various diseases, including multiple myeloma, pancreatic cancer, myelodysplastic syndromes, colon cancer, psoriasis, and Alzheimer's disease.

Curcumin and its related compounds have been shown to regulate bone homeostasis *in vitro*. Curcumin has a stimulatory effect on osteoblastogenesis and a suppressive effect on osteoclastogenesis. Curcumin suppresses NF-κB activation, which is mediated through stimulation of RANKL and TNF-α in osteoclastogenesis. Oral administration of curcumin has been shown to have a restorative effect on menopausal-induced bone loss using animal models *in vivo*, suggesting a role in the prevention and treatment in osteoporosis.

Moreover, UBS109, a novel carcumin analogue, has been found to have potent effects on the stimulation of osteoblastogenesis and suppression of osteoclastogenesis. An applicative usefulness in osteoporosis treatment may be expected.

Chapter 10

Green Tea Factor Cathechin and Osteoporosis Treatment

Catechin is a flavan-3-ol, a type of natural phenol and antioxidant. It is a plant secondary metabolite. It belongs to the group of flavan-3-ols (or simply flavanols), part of the chemical family of flavonoids. The name of the catechin chemical family derives from catechu, which is the tannic juice or boiled extract of *Mimosa catechu* (*Acacia catechu*). Catechin has four diastereoisomers. The most common catechin isomer is the (+)-catechin. The other stereoisomer is (-)-catechin or ent-catechin. The most common epicatechin isomer is (-)-epicatechin. Making reference to no particular isomer, the molecule can just be called catechin. The chemical structure of (+)-catechin is shown in Figure 22.

(+)-Catechin has been found to be the most powerful scavenger (antioxidant activity) between different members of the different classes of flavonoids. Catechin exists in the form of a glycoside. Antioxidant properties can also be provided using a catechin associated with a sugar. The biosynthesis of catechin begins with a 4-hydroxycinnamoyl CoA starter unit which undergoes chain extension by the addition of three malonyl-CoAs through a PKSIII pathway. 4-Hydroxycinnamoyl CoA is biosynthesized from L-phenylalanine through the Shikimate pathway. Catechin oxygenase, a key enzyme in the degradation of catechin, is present in fungi and bacteria.

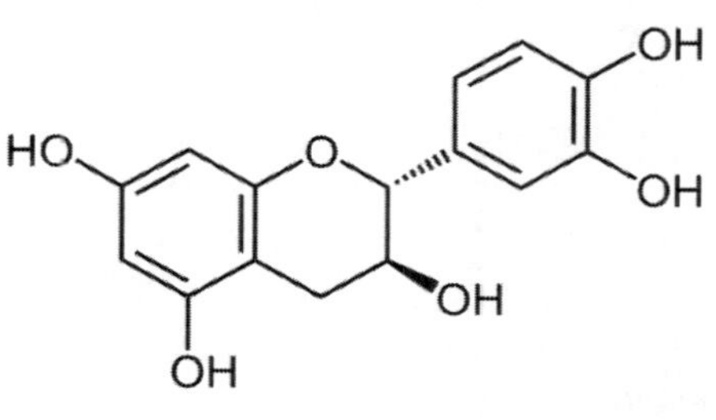

Figure 22. Chemical structure of (+)-catechin. The molecular weight of (+)-catechin ($C_{15}H_{14}O_6$) is 290.26.

(+)-Catechin and (-)-epicatechin are found in land plants such as the traditional Chinese medicine plant *Uncaria rhynchophylla*. *Potentilla fragarioides*, also used in traditional

Chinese medicine, contains D-catechin. (+)-Catechin is also found in the green alga *Myriophyllum spicatum*. Catechin and Epicatechin can be found in cocoa. The different other enantiomers can as well be found in chocolate where the different processes of fabrication can lead to epimerisation by heating. The kola nut, a related species, contains epicatechin and D-catechin. Açaí oil, obtained from the fruit of the açaí palm (*Euterpe oleracea*), is rich in (+)-catechin. (-)-Epicatechin and (+)-catechin are along the main natural phenols in argan oil. It is one of the major phenolic compounds identified in peach. Catechin is also found in vinegar.

Bioavailability of Catechin

Catechin is absorbed into intestinal cells and metabolized extensively because no native catechin can be detected in plasma from the mesenteric vein. Mesenteric plasma contains glucuronide conjugates of catechin and 3'-O-methyl catechin (3'OMC), indicating the intestinal origin of these conjugates. Additional methylation and sulfation occur in the liver, and glucuronide or sulfate conjugates of 3'OMC are excreted extensively in the bile. The concentrations of catechin derivatives in the liver are lower than in the plasma, and no accumulation is observed when the rats are adapted for 14 days to the supplemented diets. The hepatic metabolites are intensively methylated (90–95%), but in contrast to the plasma, some free aglycones can be detected. Circulating forms are mainly glucuronide conjugates of catechin and 3'OMC. Another study shows that catechin undergoes enzymatic oxidation by tyrosinase in the presence of glutathione (GSH) to form mono-, bi-, and tri-glutathione conjugates of catechin and mono- and bi-glutathione conjugates of a catechin dimer. In human, (+)-catechin absorbed orally is metabolized largely within 24 hours with the production of eleven metabolites detected in the urine.

Biological Effects of Catechin

Catechin reduces atherosclerotic lesion development in apo E-deficient mice, and it has stereospecific opposite effects on glycogen metabolism in isolated rat hepatocytes. (+)-Catechin inhibits intestinal tumor formation in mice and the oxidation of low density lipoprotein. (+)-Catechin is a histidine decarboxylase inhibitor and inhibits the conversion of histidine to histamine, and, so, is thought to be beneficial through reduction of potentially damaging, histamine-related local immune response(s).

(+)-Catechin and (-)-epicatechin are also selective monoamine oxidase inhibitors (MAOIs) of type MAO-B, which may be used to reduce the symptoms of Parkinson's and Alzheimer's patients. The catechin family of compounds is strong therapeutic candidates for protection against the cognitive decline caused by HIV. Epicatechin, epigallocatechin gallate (EGCG) and other catechin flavonoids may protect against neurotoxic oxidative stress caused by the HIV-Tat protein. Epicatechin is able to cross the blood-brain barrier more efficiently than resveratrol, which is more hydrophilic. LD_{50} for (+)-catechin is shown to be 10,000 mg/kg body weight in rat and mice.

Effects of Catechin in Bone Homeostasis

Effect of Catechin on Osteoblastogenesis

Green tea has been reported to possess antioxidant, antitumorigenic, and antibacterial qualities that regulate the endocrine system. Various physiological effects of the tea polyphenol catechin for alleviating diseases such as cancer, arteriosclerosis, hyperlipidaemia and osteoporosis have been shown. Previous epidemiological studies found that the bone mineral density (BMD) of postmenopausal women with a habit of tea drinking was higher than that of women without habitual tea consumption. However, the effects of green tea catechins on osteogenic function have rarely been investigated.

The direct effects of this flavonoid on bone mineralization have been investigated. Tumor necrosis factor-α (TNF-α) and interleukin-6 (IL-6) are candidate cytokines which are produced by osteoblastic linage cells and promote osteoblast apoptosis, osteoclastogenesis, and bone resorption. The effect of (+)-catechin, one of the most common grape flavonols, on osteoblastic MC3T3-E1 cells has been reported [347]. (+)-Catechin caused a significant elevation of cell survival at 10^{-5} and 10^{-4} M and alkaline phosphatase activity at 10^{-5} M. Also, treatment with (+)-catechin (10^{-5} M) decreased bone-resorbing cytokines (TNF-α and IL-6) production and apoptosis in osteoblasts [347]. These observations suggest that the reduction of bone-resorbing cytokines and apoptosis in osteoblasts by (+)-catechin may result in the prevention and therapy for osteoporosis and inflammatory bone diseases [347].

Consumption of green tea, a rich source of epigallocatechin-3-gallate (EGCG), is associated with increased bone mineral density. Moreover, it has been examined whether EGCG [(-)-epigallocatechin-3-gallate], which is the main component of green tea catechin, has a physiologic effect on osteoblast development using the precursor cell line of osteoblasts, MC3T3-E1, and co-culture of the osteoblasts from mouse newborn calvaria and mouse bone marrow cells [348]. Although EGCG did not affect the viability and proliferation of MC3T3-E1 cells, EGCG inhibited the osteoblast differentiation [348]. EGCG did not affect the mineralization of differentiated MC3T3-E1 cells, and reduced osteoclast formation in co-culture [348]. These results suggest that EGCG can effectively suppress bone resorption, and can be used as an effective medicine in the treatment of the symptoms of osteoporosis.

The effects of EGCG on the formation of mineralized bone nodules by SaOS-2 human osteoblast-like cells have also been examined [349]. EGCG at concentrations of 1-5 μM caused a dose-dependent increase in the number and area of mineralized bone nodules as assessed by both von Kossa and Alizarin red staining [349]. EGCG also increased alkaline phosphatase activity, an early marker of osteoblastic differentiation [349]. After 48 hours of treatment, EGCG decreased protein levels of Runx2, a transcription factor that regulates osteoblast maturation by inhibiting late-stage differentiation [349]. The observed effects of EGCG on bone formation by human osteoblast-like cells suggest that EGCG may have beneficial effects on bone health.

It has been revealed that triiodothyronine (T3)-activated p38 mitogen-activated protein (MAP) kinase, but not p44/p42 MAP kinase, is involved in the synthesis of osteocalcin in osteoblast-like MC3T3-E1 cells [350]. EGCG significantly suppressed T3-stimulated osteocalcin synthesis [350]. The inhibitory effect of EGCG was dose-dependent in the range of 3 to 30 μM. On the other hand, T3-induced phosphorylation of p38 MAP kinase was not affected by EGCG [350]. EGCG profoundly inhibited T3-stimulated transcriptional activity [350]. These results strongly suggest that EGCG suppresses T3-stimulated osteocalcin synthesis upstream of the transcriptional level in osteoblast-like MC3T3-E1 cells [350].

Moreover, the effects of EGCG on cell proliferation, the mRNA expressions of relevant osteogenic markers, alkaline phosphatase (ALP) activity and mineralization have been examined [351]. In a murine bone marrow mesenchymal stem cell line, D1, the mRNA expressions of core binding factors a1 (Cbfa1/Runx2), osterix, osteocalcin, ALP increased after 48 hours of EGCG treatment [351]. ALP activity was also significantly augmented upon EGCG treatment for 4, 7 and 14 days [351]. Furthermore, mineralizations assayed by Alizarin Red S and von Kossa stain were enhanced after EGCG treatment for 2-4 weeks in D1 cell cultures [351]. However, a 24-hour treatment of EGCG inhibited thymidine incorporation of D1 cells [351]. These observations demonstrate that long-term treatment of EGCG increases the expressions of osteogenic genes, elevates ALP activity and eventually stimulates mineralization, in spite of its inhibitory effect on proliferation. This suggests that the stimulatory effects of EGCG on osteogenesis of mesenchymal stem cells may be one of the mechanisms that allow tea drinkers to possess higher BMD [351].

As described above, EGCG may have an effect on osteoblastogenesis *in vitro*.

Effects of Catechin in Osteoclastogenesis

A pretreatment with (+)-catechin renders embryonic mouse calvaria in culture resistant to the action of bone resorbing agents, either parathyroid hormone (PTH), prostaglandin E_2 or retinoic acid, and inhibits in a parallel way the enhanced excretion of N-acetyl-beta-glucosaminidase, a reference lysosomal enzyme, induced by these agents; it has, however, no effect on the small spontaneous leakage of lactate dehydrogenase from the explants [352]. Moreover, the resorption induced in calvaria by a pretreatment with PTH or retinoic acid was inhibited by a further culture with catechin. This inhibition of bone resorption is discussed in relation with the collagen-stabilizing properties of (+)-catechin [352].

Three tea catechins, epigallocatechin (EGC), gallocatechin (GC), and gallocatechin gallate (GCG), have been investigated for their effects on bone metabolism [353]. The effects of the tea catechins on bone formation were evaluated using cultured rat osteoblast-like osteosarcoma cell line UMR-106. EGC significantly stimulated alkaline phosphatase activity at concentrations of 10 and 20 μM. The amount of mineralization also increased significantly with EGC [353]. On another cell culture platform, EGC significantly inhibited osteoclast formations from RAW 264.7 cells upon receptor activation of nuclear factor-κB ligand induction on the fourth day of treatment, at a concentration of 10 μM [353]. EGC also dose-dependently inhibited the mRNA expression of tatrate-resistant acid phosphatase. GC and GCG could decrease osteoclastogenesis at 20 μM [353]. The tea catechins, EGC in particular, may have positive effects on bone metabolism through a double process of promoting osteoblastic activity and inhibiting osteoclast differentiations.

Alveolar bone resorption is a characteristic feature of periodontal diseases and involves removal of both the mineral and the organic constituents of the bone matrix, a process mainly carried out by multinucleated osteoclast cells. (-)-Epigallocatechin gallate (EGCG), the main constituent of green tea polyphenols, has been reported to induce the apoptotic cell death of osteoclasts and to modulate caspase activation in various tumor cells. The effects of EGCG on osteoclast survival and osteoclast apoptosis via caspase activation have been examined [354]. The effect of EGCG on osteoclast survival was determined by tartrate-resistant acid phosphatase (TRAP) staining in osteoclasts differentiated from RAW 264.7 cells. In addition, the apoptosis of osteoclasts by EGCG using a DNA-fragmentation assay was assayed [354]. Involvement of caspase in EGCG-mediated osteoclast apoptosis was evaluated by treatment with a general caspase inhibitor, Z-VAD-FMK [354]. Moreover, the effect of EGCG on the activation of caspase-3 was assessed by a colorimetric activity assay and western blotting. EGCG significantly inhibited, in a dose-dependent manner, the survival of osteoclasts differentiated from RAW 264.7 cells and induced the apoptosis of osteoclasts [354]. Treatment with EGCG resulted in DNA fragmentation and induced the activation of caspase-3 in RAW 264.7 cell-derived osteoclasts [354]. Additional treatment with Z-VAD-FMK suppressed these effects of EGCG [354]. From these findings, it has been suggested that EGCG might prevent alveolar bone resorption by inhibiting osteoclast survival through the caspase-mediated apoptosis [354].

The gram-negative bacterium, Porphyromonas gingivalis has been reported to stimulate the activity and expression of several groups of matrix metalloproteinases (MMPs), whereas (-)-epigallocatechin gallate (EGCG), the main constituent of green tea polyphenols, has been reported to have inhibitory effects on the activity and expression of MMPs. The effects of the green tea polyphenol, EGCG, on the gene expression of osteoblast-derived MMP-2, -9 and -13, stimulated by P. gingivalis, and on the formation of osteoclasts have been determined [355]. The effect of EGCG on the gene expression of MMPs was examined by treating mouse calvarial primary osteoblastic cells with EGCG (20 microM) in the presence of sonicated P. gingivalis extracts. The transcription levels of MMP-2, -9 and -13 were assessed by reverse transcription-polymerase chain reaction (RT-PCR). The effect of EGCG on osteoclast formation was confirmed by tartrate-resistant acid phosphatase (TRAP) staining in a co-culture system of mouse bone marrow cells and calvarial primary osteoblastic cells. Treatment with the sonicated P. gingivalis extracts stimulated the expression of MMP-9 mRNA and this effect was significantly reduced by EGCG, whereas the transcription levels of MMP-2 and MMP-13 were not affected by either the sonicated P. gingivalis extracts or EGCG [355]. In addition, EGCG significantly inhibited osteoclast formation in the co-culture system at a concentration of 20 μM. These findings suggest that EGCG may prevent the alveolar bone resorption that occurs in periodontal diseases by inhibiting the expression of MMP-9 in osteoblasts and the formation of osteoclasts [355].

Matrix metalloproteinases (MMPs) play an important role in degeneration of the matrix associated with bone and cartilage. Regulation of osteoclast activity is essential in the treatment of bone disease, including osteoporosis and rheumatoid arthritis. Polyphenols in green tea, particularly epigallocatechin-3-gallate (EGCG), inhibit MMPs expression and activity. However, the effects of the black tea polyphenol, theaflavin-3, 3'-digallate (TFDG), on osteoclast and MMP activity are unknown. Therefore, it has been examined whether TFDG and EGCG affect MMP activity and osteoclast formation and differentiation *in vitro* [356]. TFDG or EGCG (10 and 100 μM) was added to cultures of rat osteoclast precursor cells and mature osteoclasts. Numbers of multinucleated osteoclasts and actin rings decreased in polyphenol-treated cultures relative to control cultures. MMP-2 and MMP-9 activities were lower in TFDG- and EGCG-treated rat osteoclast precursor cells than in control cultures [356]. MMP-9 mRNA levels declined significantly in TFDG-treated osteoclasts in comparison to control osteoclasts [356]. TFDG and EGCG inhibited the formation and differentiation of osteoclasts via inhibition of MMPs [356]. TFDG may suppress actin ring formation more effectively than EGCG. Thus, TFDG and EGCG may be suitable agents or lead compounds for the treatment of bone resorption diseases.

EGCG has been shown to suppress osteoclast differentiation. However, the precise molecular mechanisms underlying the inhibitory action of EGCG in osteoclastogenesis and the effect of EGCG on inflammation-mediated bone destruction remain unclear. Moreover, it has been found that EGCG inhibited osteoclast formation induced by osteoclastogenic factors in bone marrow cell-osteoblast cocultures but did not affect the ratio of receptor activator of nuclear factor κB (NF-κB) ligand (RANKL) to osteoprotegerin induced by osteoclastogenic factors in osteoblasts [357]. It was also found that EGCG inhibited osteoclast formation from bone marrow macrophages (BMMs) induced by macrophage colony-stimulating factor plus RANKL in a dose-dependent manner without cytotoxicity. Pretreatment with EGCG significantly inhibited RANKL-induced increase in the gene expression of c-Fos and nuclear factor of activated T-cells (NFATc1), which are essential transcription factors for osteoclast development [357]. EGCG suppressed RANKL-induced activation of c-Jun N-terminal protein kinase (JNK) pathway, among the three well known mitogen-activated protein kinases and also inhibited RANKL-induced phosphorylation of the NF-κB p65 subunit at Ser276 and NF-κB transcriptional activity without affecting the degradation of IκBalpha and NF-κB DNA-binding in BMMs [357]. The inhibitory effect of EGCG on osteoclast formation was somewhat reversed by retroviral c-Fos overexpression, suggesting that c-Fos is a downstream target for antiosteoclastogenic action of EGCG [357]. In addition, EGCG treatment reduced interleukin-1-induced osteoclast formation and bone destruction in mouse calvarial bone *in vivo*. Taken together, these obserbations suggest that EGCG has an antiosteoclastogenic effect by inhibiting RANKL-induced the activation of JNK/c-Jun and NF-κB pathways, thereby suppressing the gene expression of c-Fos and NFATc1 in osteoclast precursors.

People who regularly drink tea have been found to have a higher bone mineral density (BMD) and to be at less risk of hip fractures than those who do not drink it. Green tea catechins such as EGCG have been reported to increase osteogenic functioning in mesenchymal stem cells. Moreover, the effect of EGCG on RANKL-activation osteoclastogenesis and NF-κB in RAW 264.7, a murine preosteoclast cell line has been examined [358]. EGCG (10-100 μM) significantly suppressed RANKL-induced differentiation of osteoclasts and the formation of pits in murine RAW 264.7 cells and bone marrow macrophages (BMMs) [358]. EGCG appeared to target osteoclastic differentiation at an early stage but had no cytotoxic effect on osteoclast precursors [358]. In addition, it significantly inhibited RANKL-induced NF-κB transcriptional activity and nuclear translocation [358]. It is concluded that EGCG inhibits osteoclastogenesis through its activation of NF-κB [358].

Other study characterizes the impact of EGCG on lipopolysaccharide (LPS)-induced innate signaling in bone marrow-derived macrophages (BMMs) isolated from mice [359]. The effect of EGCG on LPS-induced pro-inflammatory gene expression and nuclear factor-κB (NF-κB) and mitogen-activated protein kinase (MAPK) signaling has been examined using reverse transcription-polymerase chain reaction, Western blotting, immunofluorescence, and the electrophoretic mobility shift assay. EGCG inhibited accumulation of LPS-induced IL-12p40, IL-6, MCP-1, ICAM-1, and VCAM-1 mRNA in BMMs [359]. EGCG blocked LPS-induced IκBα degradation and RelA nuclear translocation [359]. EGCG blocked the DNA-binding activity of NF-κB. LPS-induced phosphorylation of

ERK1/2, JNK, and p38 was inhibited by EGCG. U0126 (an inhibitor of MEK-1/2) suppressed the LPS-induced IL-12p40, IL-6, MCP-1, ICAM-1, and VCAM-1 mRNA accumulation in BMMs [359]. These findings indicate that EGCG may prevent LPS-induced pro-inflammatory gene expression through blocking NF-κB and MAPK signaling pathways in BMMs.

Thus, the suppressive effects of EGCG on osteoclastogenesis and bone resorption are elucidated at molecular levels.

Role of Dietary Catechin in Osteoporosis Treatment

Recent studies have suggested that green tea polyphenols are promising agents for preventing bone loss in women. Findings that green tea polyphenols supplementation resulted in increased urinary green tea polyphenols concentrations and bone mass via an increase of antioxidant capacity and/or a decrease of oxidative stress damage suggest a significant role of green tea polyphenols in bone health of women. However, the mechanism related to the possible protective role of green tea polyphenols in bone loss is not well understood. The bioavailability, mechanisms, bone mass, and safety of green tea polyphenols in preventing bone loss in middle-aged rats without (sham, SH) and with ovariectomy (OVX) have been examined [360]. A 16-week study of 2 (SH vs. OVX) x 3 (no green tea polyphenols, 0.1% green tea polyphenols, and 0.5% green tea polyphenols in drinking water) factorial design using 14-month-old female rats (n = 10/group) was performed. An additional 10 rats in baseline group were euthanized at the beginning of study to provide baseline parameters. There was no difference in femur bone mineral density between baseline and the SH+0.5% green tea polyphenols group [360]. Ovariectomy resulted in lower values for liver glutathione peroxidase activity, serum estradiol, and bone mineral density [360]. Green tea polyphenols supplementation resulted in increased urinary epigallocatechin and epicatechin concentrations, liver glutathione peroxidase activity and femur bone mineral density, decreased urinary 8-hydroxy-2'-deoxyguanosine and urinary calcium levels, but no effect on serum estradiol and blood chemistry levels [360]. It has been concluded that a bone-protective role of green tea polyphenols may contribute to an increase of antioxidant capacity and/or a decrease of oxidative stress damage [360].

It has been showed that AMP-activated protein kinase (AMPK) negatively regulates receptor activator of nuclear factor-κB ligand-induced osteoclast formation *in vitro*. Then, the effect of EGCG, an AMPK activator, on ovariectomy (OVX)-induced bone loss in mice has been shown [361]. Female mice subjected to OVX were administered EGCG for 8 weeks. Total-body bone mineral density (BMD) before and after the operation at an interval of 4 weeks was measured [361]. Micro-computed tomography (micro-CT) of the tibia and bone histomorphometric examination of the femur was also performed. Western blot analysis was additionally performed, to detect levels of the phosphorylated and total forms of AMPK-α in calvarial extracts. EGCG prevented OVX-induced body weight gain [361]. The OVX control did not show a significant increase in BMD values at baseline and after treatment, unlike the sham control [361]. EGCG attenuated OVX-induced bone loss. Micro-CT experiments revealed that EGCG induced a significant increase in trabecular bone volume and trabecular number and a decrease in trabecular spacing compared to the OVX control [361]. Histomorphometric analyses further showed that EGCG suppressed osteoclast surface and number. Phosphorylated AMPK expression was significantly elevated in bone following EGCG treatment [361]. These findings collectively indicate that EGCG decreases OVX-induced bone loss via inhibition of osteoclasts.

Bone resorption is positively regulated through receptor activator of nuclear factor-kapperB ligand (RANKL). Pro-inflammatory cytokines, such as interleukin (IL)-1β, promote RANKL expression by stromal cells and osteoblasts. Green tea catechin has beneficial effects on human health and has been reported to inhibit osteoclast formation in an *in vitro* co-culture system. However, there has been no investigation of the effect of green tea catechin on periodontal bone resorption *in vivo*. Therefore, it has been investigated whether green tea catechin has an inhibitory effect on lipopolysaccharide (LPS)-induced bone resorption [362]. Escherichia coli (E. coli) LPS or LPS with green tea catechin was injected a total of 10 times, once every 48 hours, into the gingivae of BALB/c mice. Another group of mice, housed with free access to water containing green tea catechin throughout the experimental period, were also injected with LPS in a similar manner. The alveolar bone resorption and IL-1β expression induced by LPS in gingival tissue were significantly decreased by injection or oral administration of green tea catechin [362]. Furthermore, when green tea catechin was added to the medium, decreased responses to LPS were observed in CD14-expressing Chinese hamster ovary (CHO) reporter cells, which express CD25 through LPS-induced nuclear factor-kappaB (NF-κB) activation [362]. These findings demonstrate that green tea catechin inhibits nuclear translocation of NF-κB activated by LPS. In addition, osteoclasts were generated from mouse bone marrow macrophages cultured in a medium containing RANKL and macrophage colony-stimulating factor with or without green tea catechin. The number of osteoclasts was decreased in dose-dependent manner when green tea catechin was added to the culture medium [362]. These observaqtions suggest that green tea catechin suppresses LPS-induced bone resorption by inhibiting IL-1β production or by directly inhibiting osteoclastogenesis.

Postmenopausal estrogen deficiency often causes bone density loss and osteoporosis. The effects of an oral administration of oil palm leaf extract (OPL) on bone calcium content and structure, bone density, ash weights, and serum total alkaline phosphatase (T-ALP) of estrogen-deficient ovariectomized (OVX) rats have been examined [363]. Female Sprague-Dawley rats were divided into five experimental groups: 1) intact (normal control); 2) ovariectomized (OVX control), and OVX rats supplemented with 3) 2% (w/v) green tea (OVX + GT), 4) oil palm leaf extract 150 mg/kg of body weight, or 5) oil palm leaf extract 300 mg/kg of body weight in the drinking water. After 3 months, the OVX control rats had significantly decreased femur and tibia masses (-5% and -3%, respectively), ash (-15% and -10%), calcium content (-0.5% and -2.7%), and bone density and T-ALP concentrations (-40%) compared with intact rats. The catechin-rich oil palm leaf extract dose dependently increased the OVX bone density and structure, femur and tibia masses (by +8% and +12% respectively), ash (by +30% and +20% respectively), calcium (by +3% and +5%), and T-ALP concentrations (by +76%) compared with the OVX rats [363]. The increases by oil palm leaf extract were higher than that in OVX + GT and control intact rats [363].The catechin-rich oil palm leaf extract increased the bone mass in estrogen-deficient rats by increasing osteoblast activities to higher levels than in normal rats and those supplemented with GT [363]. This was shown by the modulation of serum T-ALP levels, bone calcium content, total mineral content, and bone histologic structure. The oil palm leaf extract may be a potential inexpensive ingredient for protection against osteoporosis and influences bone metabolism by encouraging bone formation [363].

Conclusion

Consumption of green tea, a rich source of epigallocatechin-3-gallate (EGCG), is associated with increased bone mineral density, suggesting a role in the prevention of osteoporosis. EGCG has been demonstrated to have stimulatory effects on osteoblastogenesis and mineralization and suppressive effects on osteoclastogenesis and bone resorption *in vitro*. EGCG regulates the gene expression of various proteins which are involved in osteoblastogenesis and osteoclastogenesis. Supplementation of green tea extract and EGCG prevented bone loss induced in ovariectomized rats *in vivo*, supporting the view that dietary EGCG may be useful in the prevention and treatment of osteoporosis.

Chapter 11

Plant Product Honokiol and Bone Homeostasis

Magnolia officinalis, a component of Asian herbal teas, has long been employed in traditional Japanese and Chinese medicine to treat numerous maladies. Honokiol, a biphenolic compound, is now considered to be one of the major active ingredients of *Magnolia* extract, and is under intense investigation for its anti-angiogenic, anti-inflammatory, antitumor and neuroprotective properties.

Honokiol, a neolignan, is a physiologically active component of kouboku (*Magnolia obovata*) and is a phenolic compound isolated from the bark of *Magnolia officinalis.* Chemical structure of honokiol is shown in Figure 23. Honokiol is a lignan, which is present in the cones, bark, and leaves of *Magnolia grandiflora* that has been used in the traditional Japanese medicine *Saiboku-to* as an anxiolytic, antithrombotic, antidepressant, antiemetic, and antibacterial. While early research on the effective compounds in traditional remedies has simply used whole magnolia bark extracts, known as houpu *magnolia*, recent study has identified honokiol and its structural isomer magnolol as the active compounds in *magnolia* bark. In the late 1990s, honokiol saw a revival in Western countries as a potent and highly tolerable antitumorigenic and neurotrophic compound.

Biological Effects of Honokiol

Honokiol has been shown to have pro-apoptotic effects in melanoma, sarcoma, myeloma, leukemia, bladder, lung, prostate, oral squamous cell carcinoma and colon cancer cell lines, suggesting its anti-tumorigenic activity. Honokiol inhibits phosphorylation of Akt, p44/42 mitogen-activated protein kinase (MAPK), and src. Additionally, honokiol regulates the nuclear factor kappa B (NF-κB) activation pathway, an upstream effector of vascular endothelial growth factor (VEGF), MCL1, and cyclooxygenase 2 (COX-2), all significant pro-angiogenic and survival factors. Honokiol induces caspase-dependent apoptosis in a TRAIL-mediated manner, and potentiates the pro-apoptotic effects of doxorubicin and other etoposides. So potent is honokiol's pro-apoptotic effects that it overcomes even notoriously drug resistant neoplasms such as multiple myeloma and chronic B-cell leukemia.

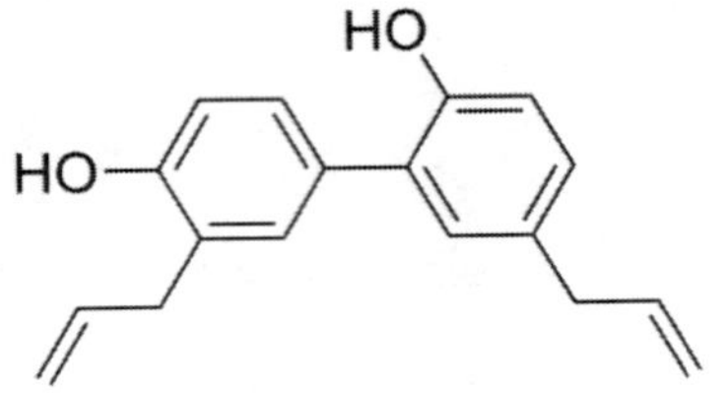

Figure 23. Chemical structure of honokiol. The molecular weight of honokiol ($C_{18}H_{18}O_2$) is 266.33.

Honokiol has also been shown to promote neurite outgrowth and have neuroprotective effects in rat cortical neurons. Additionally, honokiol increases free cytoplasmic Ca^{2+} in rat cortical neurons. Honokiol is a weak cannabinoid CB2 receptor ligand but the naturally occurring derivative 4-O-methylhonokiol was shown to be a potent and selective cannabinoid CB2 receptor inverse agonist and to possess antiosteoclastic effects.

In addition, honokiol inhibits platelet aggregation in rabbits in a dose-dependent manner, and protects cultured RAEC against oxidized low density lipoprotein injury. Honokiol significantly increases the prostacyclin metabolite 6-keto-PGF1alpha, potentially the key factor in honokiol's anti-thrombotic activity. Honokiol is known to act on the $GABA_A$ receptors.

Effects of Honokiol in Bone Homeostasis

Skeletal renewal is a delicate balance between bone resorbing osteoclasts and bone forming osteoblasts. The effects of honokiol in bone homeostasis have been found. There has been a strong interest in searching for natural therapies for osteoporosis. The effects of honokiol on the function of osteoblastic MC3T3-E1 cells have been examined [364]. Honokiol caused a significant elevation of cell growth, alkaline phosphatase activity, collagen synthesis, mineralization, glutathione content, and osteoprotegerin release in the cells [364]. Moreover, honokiol significantly decreased the production of osteoclast differentiation inducing factors such as TNF-α, IL-6, and receptor activator of nuclear factor-κB ligand (RANKL) in the presence of antimycin A, which inhibits mitochondrial electron transport and has been used as a reactive oxygene species generator. These findings suggest that honokiol may have positive effects on skeletal structure.

Osteoclasts form from precursors that circulate among the monocyte lineage and differentiation into osteoclasts under the influence of the key osteoclastogenic cytokine receptor activation of NF-κB ligand (RANKL) [7-9]. It has been investigated whether honokiol has effects on the differentiation and function of osteoclasts induced by RANKL [365]. Honokiol markedly inhibited RANKL-induced tartrate-resistant acid phosphatase (TRAP) activity and the formation of TRAP-positive multinucleated cells in both bone marrow-derived monocytes and RAW264 cells [365]. In experiments to elucidate its mechanism of action, honokiol was found to suppress RANKL-induced phosphorylation of p38 mitogen-activated protein kinase (MAPK), extracellular signal-regulated kinase (ERK), and c-Jun N-terminal kinase (JNK). The RANKL-induced expressions of c-Fos and nuclear factor of activated T cells-c1 (NFATc1), which are crucial transcriptional factors for osteoclastogenesis, were also reduced by treatment with honokiol [365]. Furthermore, honokiol induced disruption of the actin rings in mature osteoclasts without affecting the cell viability and suppressed osteoclastic pit formation on dentin slices [365]. Taken together, these findings suggest that honokiol inhibits osteoclast differentiation by suppressing the activation of MAPKs (p38 MAPK, ERK and JNK), decreasing the expressions of c-Fos and NFATc1, and attenuates bone resorption by disrupting the actin rings in mature osteoclasts. Therefore, honokiol could prove useful for the treatment of bone diseases associated with excessive bone resorption.

Honokiol Stimulates Osteoblastogenesis by Suppressing Nf-κB Activation

Honokiol is a small-molecule polyphenol isolated from the genus *Magnolia* and has been found to have anti-angiogenic, anti-inflammatory, and anti-tumor properties in preclinical models, with low toxicity [366]. Biochemically, honokiol has been recognized to regulate NF-κB signaling and to block TNF-α-induced NF-κB activation, IkBα phosphorylation, and IkBα degradation [366].

Activation of the NF-κB signal transduction pathway by RANKL is an essential step in osteoclast differentiation and function [9] and pharmacological antagonists of NF-κB activation repress osteoclastogenesis *in vitro* [229] and bone resorption *in vivo* [290]. By contrast, activation of NF-κB signaling by inflammatory cytokines such as TNF-α potently inhibits osteoblast differentiation and function *in vitro* [9] and *in vivo* [290]. By contrast, suppression of NF-κB promotes osteoblast differentiation and mineralization *in vitro* [290, 292, 293] and bone formation at baseline [290] and in *in vivo* models of estrogen deficiency [289] and of fracture repair [287].

Consistent with this anti-NF-κB activity, honokiol was found to inhibit RANKL-induced osteoclastogenesis *in vitro* [367] to inhibit the progression of collagen-induced arthritis (an animal model of the inflammatory autoimmune disease and rheumatoid arthritis) *in vivo*, by downregulating inflammatory cytokines, matrix metalloproteinases and blocking oxidative tissue damage [368].

Given the capacity of honokiol to antagonize NF-κB activation, it has been examined whether honokiol promotes osteoblast differentiation and mineralization *in vitro*. Honokiol may indeed have significant potential for use as a bone anabolic agent [369]. Honokiol has been found to augment the differentiation of osteoblastic MC3T3 into mineralizing osteoblasts and alleviates the suppressive effect of TNF-α on osteoblast mineralization [369].

To investigate the effect of honokiol on *in vitro* osteoblast differentiation and activity, the author *et al.* treated osteoblastic MC3T3 cells with honokiol (1, 10 or 100 μM) in mineralizing medium for 18 days and stained for calcium deposition with Alizarin Red-S [369]. The data showed that at 1 and 10 μM honokiol augmented the differentiation of osteoblastic MC3T3 cells into mineralizing osteoblasts [369]. At 100 μM, mineralization was inhibited, although cells were still alive and attached to the plate [369].

TNF-α is an established inhibitor of osteoblastic differentiation both *in vivo* and *in vitro* [284, 290]. Consistent with these known actions, TNF-α (5 ng/ml) suppressed mineralization of osteoblastic MC3T3 cells [369]. Addition of honokiol at 0.1 μM and above alleviated the repressive effect of TNF-α and potentiated mineralization [369].

Honokiol suppressed basal and TNF-α-induced NF-κB activity in osteoblastic MC3T3 cells [369]. Because honokiol has been reported to antagonize NF-κB, a pathway inhibitory to osteoblast differentiation and a key mechanism of TNF-α signaling whether honokiol antagonizes basal and/or TNF-α-induced NF-κB activation was investigated using transiently transfected osteoblastic MC3T3 cells with an NF-κB luciferase reporter and quantitated luciferase activity in the presence or absence of honokiol [369]. Honokiol weakly, but significantly, suppressed basal NF-κB activity and potently and dose-dependently (0.1 to 100 μM) suppressed TNF-α-induced NF-κB activity [369].

Honokiol may antagonize the nuclear accumulation of p65 NF-κB subunit by TNF-α and promotes cytosolic retention of IκBα [369]. The NF-κB subunit p65 is considered to be a major species in osteoblasts, and Western blots for p65 on nuclear and cytosolic extracts from MC3T3 osteoblast precursors, in the presence or absence of TNF-α and/or honokiol was performed. Honokiol was found to markedly reduce basal and TNF-α-induced p65 nuclear translocation [369]. Consistent with these data honokiol promoted cytosolic retention of IκBα under basal conditions as well as following TNFα stimulation [369].

Honokiol has been recognized as an antagonist of NF-κB activation in a number of cell types, and consistent with such action has been reported to inhibit osteoclast differentiation [367], an NF-κB-dependent proces. TNF-α, a potent inducer of NF-κB has been previously to be reported a suppressor of bone formation *in vivo*, and in mice and even at physiological concentrations significantly lowers peak attainable bone mineral density (BMD) [290].

The reverse process however, NF-κB suppression, promotes osteoblast differentiation *in vitro* by pharmacological antagonists [290] as well as by nutritional factors with bone anabolic properties including vitamin K_2 [229], and the carotenoids *p*-hydroxycinnamic acid and β-cryptoxanthin [293]. Honokiol, which reveals virtue of its anti-NF-κB activity, was also demonstrated to possess bone anabolic activity. The author *et al.* tested this notion *in vitro*, and found that honokiol does indeed upregulate mineralization by the preosteoblastic cell line MC3T3, as well as reversing the suppressive action of TNF-α on mineralization. Honokiol further suppressed NF-κB activation in the context of a biological assay (the NF-κB-driven reporter system) demonstrating a potent and sustained effect [369]. Consistent with the bio-assay, it was found that nuclear translocation of the NF-κB subunit p65 was suppressed by honokiol and that the cytosolic concentration of the physiological NF-κB activation inhibitor IκB, was intensified following treatment by honokiol [369]. These findings were consistent with previous findings showing that honokiol inhibits TNF-α-induced NF-κB activation, and IkBα degradation [366].

Honokiol alleviated the suppressive actions of TNF-α on BMP-2- and TGF-β-induced Smad activation in MC3T3 cells [369]. TNF-α suppresses osteoblast differentiation in part by antagonizing Smad activation by bone morphogenetic proteins (BMP) including BMP-2 and early osteoblast commitment factor TGF-β [369]. We thus examined the effect of honokiol on basal, BMP-2-induced and TGF-β-induced Smad activation and the capacity of honokiol to reverse the suppressive action of TNF-α on Smad induction by BMP-2 and TGF-β using a Smad-luciferase reporter responsive to all Smad species [290]. While honokiol had no direct effect on basal, BMP-2-, or TGF-β-induced Smad-activation it significantly reversed the suppressive activity of TNF-α on BMP-2 and TGF-β induced Smad activation [369].

TGF-β is an early osteoblast commitment factor [324] and induces migration of bone mesenchymal stem cells (osteoblast precursors) to sites of bone turnover [370]. BMPs by contrast, are potent inducers of osteoblast differentiation. Both TGF-β and BMPs are potent inducers of Smad signaling, although TGF-β uses predominantly R-Smads 2 and 3, while BMPs promote mainly R-Smads 1, 5, and 8. One mechanism by which TNF-α suppresses osteoblast differentiation is through NF-κB-mediated antagonism of TGF-β- and BMP-2-induced Smad signaling in differentiating osteoblasts [290]. Other studies have further reported that NF-κB signaling in osteoblasts upregulates the inhibitor of Smad-signaling, Smad7 [291], and that TNF-α promoting proteasomal degradation of BMP signaling proteins by upregulating Smad ubiquitination regulatory factor 1 (Smurf1), a process that leads to systemic bone loss [340]. NF-κB antagonists including the a pharmacological peptide based on the Nemo Binding Domain [290] and vitamin K_2 [229] can alleviate this repressive action of TNF-α on Smad signaling. Honokiol too may possess this ability.

NF-κB antagonists may represent novel dual anabolic and anti-catabolic drugs. Honokiol may represent one such agent. A significant advantage of honokiol over biologics that require injection is its demonstrated bioavailability following oral delivery in animal models [369]. Furthermore, as honokiol is a simple polyphenol compound, it can be synthesized in large concentrations at low cost. Honokiol may have significant potential for development into a bone anabolic agent for amelioration of bone loss in multiple metabolic disease states. Studies in animal models are now needed to demonstrate bone anabolic activity of honokiol *in vivo*.

Effect of Honokiol on Bone Metastasis

Honokiol, a soluble nontoxic natural product derived from *Magnolia*, has been shown to induce apoptosis in malignant cells. The effect of honokiol and the combined therapy with docetaxel on prostate cancer growth and bone metastasis has been investigated in experimental models [371]. The *in vitro* proapoptotic effects of honokiol on human androgen-dependent and -independent prostate cancer, bone marrow, bone marrow-derived endothelial, and prostate stromal cells have been examined. Honokiol-induced activation of caspases was evaluated by Western blot and FACS analysis. To confirm the cytotoxicity of honokiol, mice bone was inoculated *in vivo* with androgen-independent prostate cancer, C4-2 cells and the effects of honokiol and/or docetaxel on prostate cancer growth in bone were evaluated. Daily honokiol (100 mg/kg) and/or weekly docetaxel (5 mg/kg) were intraperitoneally injected for 6 weeks [371]. Prostate cancer growth in mouse bone was evaluated by radiography, serum prostate-specific antigen (PSA) and tissue immunohistochemistry. Honokiol induced apoptosis in all cell lines tested [371]. In prostate cancer cells, honokiol induced apoptosis via the activation of caspases 3, 8, and 9 and the cleavage of poly-adenosine diphosphate ribose polymerase in a dose- and time-dependent manner [371]. Honokiol was shown to inhibit the growth and depress serum PSA in mice harboring C4-2 xenografts in the skeleton and the combination with docetaxel showed additive effects that inhibited further growth without evidence of systemic toxicity [371]. Immunohistochemical staining confirmed honokiol exhibited growth-inhibitory, apoptotic, and antiangiogenic effects on prostate cancer xenografts. The combination of honokiol and low-dose docetaxel may be used to improve patient outcome in androgen-independent prostate cancer with bone metastasis. Honokiol may suppress cancer cell bone metastasis-induced osteolysis, since this compound has stimulatory effects on osteoblastic bone formation and suppressive effects on osteoclastic bone resorption *in vitro*.

Conclusion

Magnolia officinalis, a component of Asian herbal teas, has long been employed in traditional Japanese and Chinese medicine to treat numerous maladies. Honokiol, a biphenolic compound, is now considered to be one of the major active ingredients of *Magnolia* extract, and is under intense investigation for its anti-angiogenic, anti-inflammatory, antitumor and neuroprotective properties. Honokiol has also been shown to have stimulatory effects on osteoblastogenesis and mineralization and suppressive effects on osteoclastogenesis *in vitro*. The adiministration of honokiol has been demonstrated to suppress prostate cancer cell bone metastasis in mice *in vivo*, suggesting that honokiol has an inhibitory effect on cancer cell bone metastasis-induced osteolysis. In addition, honokiol may be expected to have effects in the prevention and treatment of osteoporosis.

Chapter 12

Role of Marine Alga *sargassum horneri* Component in Osteoporosis Treatment

The effect of marine algae on bone metabolism has been determined in recent studies. *Undaria pinnatifida, Sargassum horneri, Eisenia bicyclis, Cryptonemia scmitziana, Gelidium amansii,* and *Ulva pertusa* Kjellman are used as food materials in Japan. Among these marine algae, *Sargassum horneri (S. horneri)* has been found to have a unique anabolic effect on bone components [372]. *S. horneri* extract has been found to have a stimulatory effect on osteoblastic bone formation and an inhibitory effect on osteoclastic bone resorption *in vitro*, thereby increasing bone mass. The intake of *S. horneri* extract caused preventive effects on bone loss in animal models for osteoporosis and in healthy human. *S. horneri* extracts may be useful as an osteogenic factor in the prevention of osteoporosis in human subjects.

This chapter has been written to outline the findings concerning the anabolic effect of *S. horneri* extract on bone metabolism and will discuss the usefulness of this functional food factor in the prevention of osteoporosis.

S. Horneri Extract Stimulates Osteoblastic Bone Formation

Preparation of *S. Horneri* Extract

Marine algae *S. horneri* [*Sargassum horneri* (Turner) C. Agardh] was seasonally gathered from the coast at Shimoda (Shizuoka Prefecture, Japan) and Miyako (Iwate Prefecture, Japan), and it was freeze-dried and powered [372]. The gathered fresh marine algae were homogenized in distilled water and are centrifuged at 5500 g in a refrigerated centrifuge for 10 minutes. The 5500 g supernatant fraction was pooled for freeze-drying. The powder of the water-solubilized extract was dissolved in ice-cold distilled water for use in the experiments. The water-solubilized extract from *S. horneri* was purified through the method of membrane fractionation to collect active component of various molecular weights.

S. Horneri Extract Stimulates Osteoblastogenesis

The effect of *S. horneri* extract on bone formation and mineralization has been examined using MC3T3 preosteoblastic cells *in vitro* [373]. Preosteoblastic cells were differentiated into mineralizing osteoblasts *in vitro* in the presence or absence of *S. horneri* extract in the medium containing mineralizing medium for 21 days and stained for calcium deposition with Alizarin Red-S. *S. horneri* extract (10 and 25 μg/ml) was found to potently enhance mineralization in osteoblastic MC3T3 cells [373]. *S. horneri* extract (25 - 100 μg/ml of medium) did not have a significant effect on cell number of MC3T3-E1 cells with culture. *S. horneri* extract did not appear to mediate direct toxic effects on the cultures as the cells were proliferated robustly over the culture period, and were still alive and visibly attached to the plate at the end of the experiment as compared with those of control group [373].

Bone morphogenic proteins (BMPs) such as BMP-2 are anabolic agents that signal through the Smad signaling pathway [22]. The effect of *S. horneri* extract on basal and BMP-2-induced Smad activation has been shown using a Smad 4-luciferase reporter responsive to all Smad species [373]. *S. horneri* extract did not have a direct effect on basal Smad activation. However, *S. horneri* extract (50 or 100 μg/ml) significantly enhanced Smad activation induced by BMP-2. Also, *S. horneri* extract (25 -100 μg/ml) significantly enhanced TGF-β1-induced Smad activation [373].

NF-κB activation is a potent inhibitory to osteoblast differentiation, and TNF-α-induced NF-κB activation leads to Smad suppression in MC3T3 osteoblast precursors [17, 18]. Whether *S. horneri* extract is able to prevent TNF-α-induced NF-κB activation in MC3T3 osteoblast precursors has been examined [373]. *S. horneri* extract (25 – 100 μg/ml of medium) significantly prevented TNF-α-induced NF-κB activation, although *S. horneri* extract did not have a direct effect on basal NF-κB activation.

Thus, *S. horneri* extract has been shown to stimulate osteoblastic differentiation and mineralization *in vitro*. TGF-β1- and BMP-2-induced activation of Smad signaling respectively plays an important role in the early commitment and differentiation of osteoblasts [22]. *S. horneri* extract was found to enhance BMP-2- or TGF-β1-induced Smad activation with the dose-dependency [373]. *S. horneri* extract-induced Smad enhancement may be an important to stimulate osteoblastic differentiation and mineralization.

NF-κB signaling has been shown to downregulate osteoblast differentiation [23, 24]. One major mechanism appears to involve the intersection of NF-κB with the Smad signaling pathway [23]. NF-κB signaling in osteoblasts intersects with and disrupts Smad signaling by promoting production of Smad7, an inhibitor of TGF-β- and BMP-induced R-Smad activation [25]. TNF-α further antagonizes BMP signaling by upregulating Smad ubiquitination regulatory factor 1 (Smurf1), promoting proteasomal degradation of bone morphogenetic signaling proteins [26]. Multiple suppressors of NF-κB activation are capable of rescuing the inhibitory effect of TNF-α on BMP-2 and/or TGF-β1-induced Smad activation [23]. *S. horneri* extract was found to suppress TNF-α-induced NF-κB activation in preosteoblastic MC3T3-E1 cells. Such a finding provides a possible mechanism by which *S. horneri* extract stimulates osteoblastic bone formation.

S. Horneri Extract Stimulates Mineralization in Bone Tissues

The anabolic effect of *S. horneri* extract on bone tissues has been found. Rat femoral-metaphyseal tissues were cultured in a medium containing water-solubilized extract (25 and 50 μg/ml) obtained from *U. pinnatifida, S. horneri, E. bicyclis, or C. scmitziana in vitro* [372]. Bone calcium content was significantly elevated in the presence of *S. horneri* extract (25 and 50 μg/ml). No effect was seen in the extracts of other marine algae. In addition, water suspensions (5%) of marine alga powder were orally administered once daily for 7 days. Bone calcium content was significantly increased after the adminostration of *U. pinnatifida, S. horneri, E. bicyclis, or C. scmitziana* [372]. Bone alkaline phosphatase activity was significantly increased after the administration of *S. horneri* or *G. amansii*. Thus, *S. horneri* extract has a unique anabolic effect on bone calcification *in vitro* and *in vivo*. This was the first time finding. The effects of *S. horneri* extract in increasing calcium content, alkaline phosphatase activity and deoxyribonucleic acid (DNA) content in the femoral-diaphyseal and -metaphyseal tissues *in vitro* was completely abolished in the presence of cycloheximide, an inhibitor of protein synthesis [374]. DNA may be an index of cell number in bone tissues [16, 21]. The anabolic effect of *S. horneri* extract may be resulted from newly synthesized protein components.

S. Horneri Extract Suppresses OsteoclAStic Bone Resorption

S. Horneri Extract Suppresses Osteoclastogenesis

S. horneri extract has been shown to suppress osteoclastic bone resorption. To examine the effect of *S. horneri* extract on osteoclast formation, RAW264.7 osteoclast precursors were differentiated into mature osteoclasts by stimulation with RANKL in the presence or absence of *S. horneri* extract with the dose range of 5 to 100 μg/ml of medium [373]. *S. horneri* extract had no effect on cell number of preosteoclasts (RAW267.4 cells) with culture. *S. horneri* extract (100 μg/ml) did not have a toxicity to the precursors suppressing their proliferation over 7 days of culture [373]. *S. horneri* extract (25 – 100 μg/ml) significantly suppressed osteoclast formation induced by RANKL [373].

NF-κB signal transduction pathway is essential for the generation of osteoclasts [17, 18]. The effect of *S. horneri* extract on NF-κB activation by RANKL in osteoclast precursors has been examined. RAW 264.7 cells were transfected with a NF-κB reporter and stimulated with RANKL to induce NF-κB activity in the presence or absence of *S. horneri* extract (5 – 100 μg/ml) [373]. *S. horneri* extract did not have a significant effect on basal NF-κB activity [373]. However, RANKL-induced increase in NF-κB activity was significantly blunted in the presence of *S. horneri* extract [373].

S. horneri extract with dose-dependency, which did not have cell toxicity, was found to have a suppressive effect on RANKL-stimulated osteoclastogenesis [373]. RANKL, the key osteoclastogenic cytokine, is central to formation of osteoclasts, the cells that resorb bone, through NF-κB signaling [17, 18]. *S. horneri* extract suppressed RANKL-induced NF-κB activation in osteoclast precursor cells [373]. This finding coincided with the observation that

S. horneri extract suppresses RANKL-induced osteoclastogenesis [373]. *S. horneri* extract may inhibit osteoclastogenesis through suppression of NF-κB activation.

The effect of *S. horneri* on mineralization in MC3T3-E1 cells with culture for 21 days was observed at 10 μg /ml [373]. However, the effects of *S. horneri* on Smad activity in MC3T3-E1 cells and on NF-κB activity in RAW 264.7 cells after culture for 24 hours were observed at 25 μg/ml [373]. The effects of *S. horneri* on osteoclastogenesis in RAW 264.7 cells after culture for 6 days were also revealed at 25 μg/ml [373]. The effect of *S. horneri* on osteoblastogenesis and osteoclastogenesis may be observed with lower doses in the culture for longer periods.

S. horneri Extract Suppresses Bone Resorption in Bone Tissues

The effects of *S. horneri* extract on bone resorption using femoral tissues *in vitro* have been examined [375]. Parathyroid hormone (PTH)- and prostagrandine E_2 (PGE_2) are known to induce osteoclastic bone resorption [162-164]. PTH- and PGE_2-induced decreases in bone calcium content were completely inhibited after culture with water-soublilized extracts (10, 25, and 50 μg/ml) [375]. Also, the extract completely inhibited PTH- or PGE_2-induced increase in medium glucose consumption and latic acid production by bone tissues [375]. Moreover, *S. horneri* extracts blocked PTH-induced increase in acid phosphatase activity in the diaphyseal and metaphyseal tissues [375]. These findings indicate that the water-solubilized extracts of *S. horneri* have a direct inhibitory effect on bone resorption in tissue culture *in vitro*.

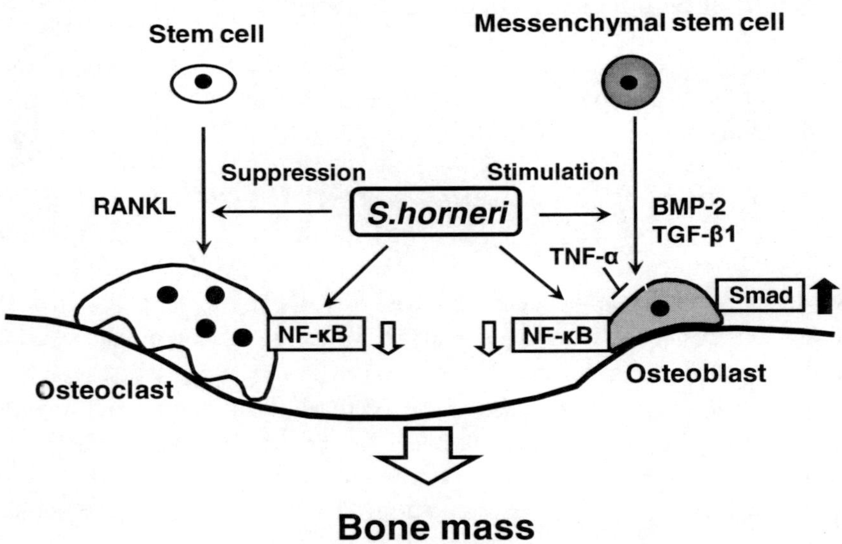

Figure 24. *S. horneri* regulates bone homeostasis. *S. horneri* component stimulates osteoblastic bone formation and suppresses osteoclastic bone resorption, thereby increasing bone mass. *S. horneri* component enhances bone growth factors (TGF-β1 and BMP-2)-induced Smad activation in osteoblasts and suppresses TNF-α- and RANL-enhanced NF-κB activation in preosteoclasts.

S. horneri extract possesses a potent Smad activation and anti-NF-κB activity and may have promise for development into an antiosteoporotic material capable of promoting new bone formation while simultaneously reducing bone resorption. *S. horneri* extract may be usefulness as a tool in the prevention of osteolysis with various pathophysiologic states. The mechanism by which *S. horneri* stimulates bone mass is summarized in Figure 24.

Characterization of Active Component in *S. horneri* Extract

As described above, *S. horneri* extracts has been found to stimulate osteoblastic bone formation [372, 373, 374] and to suppress osteoclastic bone resorption [30]. Active components, which have anabolic effects, have been found to be present in *S. horneri* extract obtained from various coasts in both Japan (Shimoda and Iwate, Japan) and China [375]. The active component of *S. horneri* extract in stimulating bone calcification has been found to be near molecular weight (MW) 3000 [375]. Meanwhile, the active component of *S. horneri* extract in inhibiting osteoclastic cell formation was less than MW 3,000 and over MW 50,000 [375, 376]. These components were stable with heat treatment. It has been speculated that the active component in stimulating bone calcification is a chemical but not peptide, and that the component over MW 50000 in inhibiting bone resorption may be a polysaccharide. These active components obtained from the coasts of Iwate (Japan) or China showed an identical molecular weight. The active component, which stimulates osteoblastogenesis and suppresses osteoclastogenesis, was found to be present in the components less than MW 3000 of *S. horneri* extract using preosteoblastic cells and RAW267.4 cells *in vitro* [373]. The active component, which stimulates osteoblastic bone formation and suppresses osteoclastic bone resorption, may be identical.

The author et al. found the existence of 4 chemicals in S. horneri components (less than MW 3000) using the analysis with liquid chromatography mass spectrophotometry system (LCMS-IT-TOF; Shimadzu, Kyoto, Japan). These chemicals were identified as 1,3,5-tris(oxolan-2-ylmethyl)-1,3,5-triazinane (MW 339), 5-phenyl-2-[2-(5-phenyltetrazol-2-yl)ethyl]tetrazole (MW 318), 3-(hexadecylamino)propane-1,2-diol (MW 316), and 2-(2-hydroxyethyl-tridecyl-amino)ethanol (MW 288). These chemicals may have an effect on osteobalstogenesis and/or osteoclastogenesis, although their biological effects on bone cells remain to be elucidated. It is possible that combination of these compounds has anabolic effects on bone.

Anabolic Effect of *S. Horneri* Extract on Bone *In Vivo*

Intake of *S. horneri* Extract Reveals Anabolic Effects on Bone

The anabolic effects of *S. horneri* extract on bone components in the femoral tissues of young and aged rats *in vivo* have been demonstrated [377]. Calcium content, alkaline phosphatase activity and DNA content in the femoral-diaphyseal and -metaphyseal tissues of young male (4-week-old) rats were significantly increased after oral administration of *S. horneri* extract (25, 50, and 100 mg/kg body weight) for 7 days [377]. Moreover, these bone components in the femoral-diaphyseal and -metaphyseal tissues of aged female (50 weeks old) rats were significantly increased after the administration of *S. horneri* extract (100 mg/kg) for 14 days, suggesting a preventive effect on bone loss with increasing age [377].

Intake of *S. horneri* Extract Suppresses Bone Loss in Diabetic State

The intake of *S. horneri* extract has been shown to have a preventive effect on bone loss in a diabetic state [378]. Diabetes has been shown to induce bone loss [299, 300]. Streptozotocin (STZ) induces decrease in insulin secretion in pancreatic cells and causes type 1 diabetes. Oral administration of *S. horneri* extract (100 mg/kg body weight) to STZ (60 mg/kg)-diabetic rats was found to have a preventive effect on bone loss with diabetes *in vivo* [378]. This finding suggests that the dietary intake of *S. horneri* extract has a preventive effect on bone loss in the pathophysiologic state. When the femoral tissues obtained from STZ-diabetic rats were cultured in medium containing *S. horneri* extract solution, the femoral calcium content and alkaline phosphatase activity were significantly increased *in vitro* [378]. Alkaline phosphatase is related to bone calcification [27, 28]. *S. horneri* extract has a stimulatory effect on bone formation [372, 374] and an inhibitory effect on bone resorption *in vitro* [375]. Presumably, the preventive effect of *S. horneri* extract on diabetes-induced bone loss may be related to a direct action of the active component of *S. horneri* extract.

Interestingly, oral administration of *S. horneri* extract (100 mg/kg) to STZ-diabetic rats has been found to have a significant preventive effect on the decrease in body weight and the increase in serum glucose and triglyceride levels induced in the diabetic state [378]. This was a novel finding. The intake of *S. horneri* extract has a partial restorative effect on serum biochemical finding with diabetes *in vivo*.

Thus, the intake of *S. horneri* extract has been demonstrated to have restorative effects on bone loss, hyperglycemia and hyperlipidemia in STZ-diabetic rats [378]. The active component of *S. horneri* extract in preventing bone loss induced with diabetic state may be identical to the component that prevents an elevation of serum glucose and triglyceride levels with diabetes.

Anabolic Effect of *S. horneri* Extract on Bone Metabolism in Human Subjects

Supplemental intake of *S. horneri* extract has been shown to have an anabolic effect on bone metabolism in human subjects [379]. Study has been undertaken to determine the effect of supplemental intake of water-solubilized *S. horneri* extract (tablets) on circulating bone metabolic markers in healthy human [379]. Thirty-six volunteers, aged 20-60 years (16 men and 20 women), were enrolled. Volunteers were divided into three groups; placebo tablet without *S. horneri* extract (5 men and 7 women), tablet containing *S. horneri* extract at 300 mg/day (6 men and 7 women) or 900 mg/day (5 men and 6 women) [379]. Placebo or *S. horneri* extract tablet was ingested once a day for 4 or 8 weeks [379]. The intake of dietary *S.*

horneri extract (900 mg/day) for 8 weeks did not have a significant alteration in other biochemical markers for the metabolic function of organs, suggesting that the intake does not have toxic effects in humans [379].

Bone-specific alkaline phosphatase [269] and γ-carboxylated osteocalcin [268] are serum bone markers of bone formation, and bone tartrate-resistant acid phosphatase (TRACP) [270] and N-telopeptides of type I collagen [271] are markers of bone resorption. Serum bone-specific alkaline phosphatase or γ-carboxylated osteocalcin concentration was not significantly changed after the intake of *S. horneri* extract (300 or 900 mg/day) for 4 or 8 weeks [379]. Serum bone tartrate-resistant acid phosphatase (TRACP) activity was significantly decreased after the intake of *S. horneri* extract (300 or 900 mg/day) for 8 weeks [379]. Serum N-telopeptides of type I collagen concentration was significantly decreased after the intake of *S. horneri* extract (900 mg/day) for 8 weeks [379]. Meanwhile, serum calcium, inorganic phosphorus and other biochemical findings were not changed after the intake of *S. horneri* extract (300 or 900 mg/day) for 4 or 8 weeks [379]. Thus, prolonged intake of *S. horneri* extract has been shown to have inhibitory effects on bone resorption in humans.

S. horneri extract has been shown to have a stimulatory effect on osteoblastic bone formation and an inhibitory effect on osteoclastic bone resorption. It has been speculated that the supplemental intake of *S. horneri* extract reveals suppressive effects on bone resorption, and later it exhibits stimulatory effects on bone formation in humans, thereby increasing bone mass. Supplemental intake of *S. horneri* extract may have effects in the prevention and treatment of bone loss with increasing age and postmenopausal women.

Conclusion

Among various marine algae which are used as food, *S. horneri* extract has been found to have a unique anabolic effect on bone mass using stimulating osteoblastic bone formation and depressing osteoclastic bone resorption due to suppressing NF-κB activation. Intake of *S. horneri* extract has usefulness in the prevention of bone loss with increasing age and diabetes. This biomedical food material may play a role in maintaining bone health and in the prevention and treatment of osteoporosis [380].

Chapter 13

Osteogenic Effect of Wasabi Leafstalk Components

Pharmacologic and nutritional factors may play a role in the prevention and treatment of bone loss with aging. Among various food and plants (including shiitake, loquat leaf, cherry leaf, gabaron tea, green tea, muskmelon, tomato, blueberry, and wasabi leafstalk), the active component to stimulate bone mineralization in mouse bone tissues *in vitro* was found to be present in the leafstalk of wasabi (*Wasabi japanica* MATSUM). The material with a low molecular weight of 158 may be the active component in wasabi leafstalk that stimulates bone mineralization. Supplemental intake of wasabi leafstalk components may have a role in the prevention and treatment of osteoporosis. The role of wasabi leafstalk components in the prevention of osteoporosis has been introduced in this chapter.

Osteogenic Factors in Wasabi Leafstalk Extracts

The effects of various foods and plants on bone tissues have been poorly understood. Then, the effects of 20% ethanol solution extracts obtained from various foods and plants on bone calcium content has been examined using mouse bone tissues *in vitro*. Among various food and plants (including shiitake, loquat leaf, cherry leaf, gabaron tea, green tea, muskmelon, tomato, blueberry, and wasabi leafstalk) used, the extracts of wasabi leafstalk (*Wasabi japanica* MATSUM) were found to have a potential anabolic effect on bone calcification in mouse calvaria tissue culture *in vitro* [347]. This was the first time finding.

Wasabi Leafstalk Extract Stimulates Bone Mineralization

Wasabi leafstalk extracts were obtained from homogenate with 20% ethanol. Culture with this extract (10 μg/ml of culture medium) caused a significant increase in calcium content and alkaline phosphatase activity, which participates in mineralization in the bone tissues [348, 349]. Wasabi leafstalk extract-induced increase in bone calcium content was completely depressed in the presence of cycloheximide, an inhibitor of protein synthesis, suggesting that the effect of wasabi leafstalk extracts is resulted from newly synthesized protein components [348]. In addition, wasabi leafstalk extract has been shown to have a suppressve effect on parathyroid hormon (PTH)-induced osteoclast-like cell formation in a mouse marrow culture system, suggesting that the component inhibits bone resorption [348]. PTH has been known to stimulate osteoclastogenesis and bone resoprtion [348].

The stimulatory effect of wasabi leafstalk extract on bone mineralization was compared with that of insulin, insulin-like growth factor-I (IGF-I), 17β-estradiol, and genistein [350]. The combination of 17β-estradiol (10^{-10} M) and wasabi leafstalk extract (15 μg/ml) had an additive effect on an increase in bone calcium content [350]. Also, the combination of either insulin (10^{-8} or 10^{-7} M) with wasabi leafstalk extract (15 μg/ml) had an additive effect an increase in bone calcium content [350]. This additive effect was not seen in case of IGF-I (10^{-8} M). Wasabi leafstalk extract enhanced anabolic effects of 17β-estradiol or insulin, which physiologically regulates bone formation *in vitro* [350].

Anabolic Effect of Wasabi Leafstalk Extract on Bone

Oral administration of wasabi leafstalk extracts to young rats cased a significant increase in alkaline phosphatase activities, calcium and DNA contents in the femoral-metaphyseal tissues (trabecullar bone) [351]. In the femoral-diaphyseal tissues (cortical bone), alkaline phosphatase activity and calcium content were increased after the administration of wasabi extract [351] This administration had a greater effect on the metaphyseal tissues than on the diaphyseal tissues [351]. Many bone cells (including chondrocytes and osteoblasts) are localized in the metaphyseal tissues. The finding, that the administration of wasabi leafstalk extract produces an increase in DNA content in the metaphyseal tissues, suggests that this administration stimulates the proliferation of bone cells. The anabolic effects of wasabi leafstalk extract on bone tissues may be based on newly synthesized protein components [351].

Whether wasabi leafstalk extracts have a preventive effect on bone loss with increasing age, which induces osteoporosis, has been examined *in vitro* and *in vivo* [352]. Bone metabolism in the femoral-diaphyseal and -metaphyseal tissues is deteriorated with increasing age (50 weeks old), as compared with that of young rats (4 weeks old) [353]. The presence of wasabi leafstalk extract in the culture medium caused a significant increase in alkaline phosphatase activity, calsium and DNA contents in the femoral-diaphyseal and -metaphyseal tissues of aged female rats *in vitro* [353]. The effect of wasabi leafstalk extract in increasing these bone components was completely depressed in the presence of an inhibitor of protein synthesis [353]. This finding suggests that the anabolic effects of wasabi leafstalk extract on bone are resulted from newly synthesized protein components in aged rat bone tissues.

Moreover, oral administration of wasabi leafstalk extract was found to induce an increase in alkaline phosphatase activity, calcium and DNA contents in the femoral-diaphyseal and -metaphyseal tissues of aged female rats *in vivo* [353]. The administration of wasabi leafstalk extract did not cause any change in body weight, serum calcium or inorganic phosphorus concentrations in aged female rats, indicating that the extract may not have a toxic effect

[353]. Thus, the intake of wasabi leafstalk extract may have a preventive effect on the deterioration of bone metabolism with increasing age. Presumably, dietary wasabi leafstalk has a preventive role in the progression of osteoporosis with aging.

Active Component of Wasabi Leafstalk Extract

The active components of wasabi leafstalk extracts that increase bone calcium content were stable when the components were treated with heat, acidity, or alkalinization [354]. The active components of wasabi leafstalk extract may not be a protein.

The active component in wasabi leafstalk has been purified [354]. Wasabi leafstalk extract was obtained from a homogenate with 20% ethanol. The active component, which was found in the ethanol extract, was purified upon gel filtration chromatography with a HiLoad 26/80 Superdex 30-pg column and reverse-phase chromatography on a Resource 15 RPC 3-ml column. The result of ESI mass spectra for the purified active component showed that the material had a molecular weight of 158 [354].

The material with a low molecular weight of 158 may be the active component in wasabi leafstalk that stimulates bone mineralization. Cinnamic acid, *p*-hydroxycinnamic acid (HCA), ferulic acid, caffeic acid or 3, 4-dimethoxycinnamic acid (DCA) has been found to be present in the wasabi leafstalk. When rat femoral tissues were cultured in a medium containing these phenolic acids, HCA was found to uniquely have an anabolic effect on bone mineralization *in vitro* [282, 283]. The molecular weight of HCA is 164. HCA is seemed to be an active component in wasabi leafstalk that reveals the anabolic effects on bone. However, it is possible that other chemical factors may be active components, because various active components may be present in wasabi leafstalk.

Conclusion

Phytochemicals, which are food functional factors, may play a role in delay degenerative bone disorders with aging and in the treatment of osteoporosis with various pathophysiological conditions. Among various food and plants (including shiitake, loquat leaf, cherry leaf, gabaron tea, green tea, muskmelon, tomato, blueberry, and wasabi leafstalk), the active component to stimulate bone mineralization in mouse bone tissues *in vitro* was found to be present in the leafstalk of wasabi (*Wasabi japanica* MATSUM) [355]. Supplemental intake of wasabi leafstalk extract has been shown to have an anabolic effect on bone metabolism in animals. Wasabi leafstalk extract may be usful in the prevention and treatment of osteoporosis.

Chapter 14

Osteogenic Effect of Bee Pollen Extract

Royal jelly, propolis and bee pollen products are commercially available, and these bee-related products are generally used as a nutrient factor. Supplemental intake of dietary bee products may help to prevent bone loss with increasing age. Among of royal jelly, propolis and bee pollen, the water-soluble extract obtained from bee pollen *Cistus ladaniferus* has been found to have anabolic effects on bone tissues *in vitro*. Bee pollen extract has stimulatory effects on osteoblastic bone formation and suppressive effects on osteoclastogenesis and bone resorption *in vitro*. Supplemental intake of bee pollen extract prevented bone loss in overiectomized and streptozotocin-induced diabetic rats *in vivo*. Bee pollen extract has been found to have an osteogenic effect and its supplemental intake may play a role in the prevention and treatment of osteoporosis.

Bee Pollen Extract Stimulates Osteoblastic Bone Formation

The effects of bee pollen, which was obtained from *Cistus ladaniferus,* on bone metabolism has not been investigated so far. This was firstly investigated by the author *et al.* [356]. Bee pollen extract was found to have anabolic effects on bone components in the femoral-diaphyseal and -metaphyseal tissues of rats *in vitro* and *in vivo* [356]. Of various bee pollens, the water-solubilized extract obtained from *Cistus ladaniferus* had a marked effect in increasing the bone calcium content. The ethanol-solubilized extract of bee pollen also was significantly increased the bone calcium content [356]. However, the effects of the extract solubilized with water in increasing the bone calcium content were greater than those of the ethnol-solubilized extract [356]. The active components in bee pollen were present in water-solubilized extract.

Culture with the extract obtained from the pollen of *C. ladaniferus* caused a significant increase in alkaline phosphatase activity and DNA content in the femoral-diaphyseal and -metaphyseal tissues *in vitro* [356]. These increases were completely inhibited in the presence of cycloheximide, suggesting that its stimulatory effect results from newly synthesized protein components.

The effect of bee pollen extract on osteoblastic MC3T3-E1 cells has been examined [357]. The water-solubilized extracts, which were obtained from the bee pollen of *Cistus ladaniferus*, were purified using the membrane fraction method with molecular weight (MW) less than 1000.

Osteoblastic cells were cultured for 72 hours in a medium containing either vehicle or bee pollen extract of less than MW 1000 (10, 25, or 50 μg/ml of medium) in the presence of 10% fetal bovine serum (FBS). The proliferation of osteoblastic cells was significantly enhanced in the presence of bee pollen extract (25 or 50 μg/ml). The stimulatory effect of bee pollen extract on cell proliferation was also observed when the cells with subconfluency were cultured for 24 or 72 hours without FBS.

Cells with sunconfluency were cultured for 24 or 72 hours in a medium containing either vehicle or bee pollen extract without FBS [357]. DNA content or alkaline phosphatase activity in osteoblastic cells was significantly increased after culture with bee pollen extract (50 μg/ml) for 24 hours [357]. The effect of 25 μg/ml of bee pollen extract on these components was seen after culture for 72 hours. This study demonstrates that the fraction of bee pollen extract of less than MW1000 has anabolic effects in osteoblastic MC3T3-E1 cells which involve in bone formation.

Bee Pollen Extract Suppresses Osteoclastic Bone Resorption

The water-solubilized extract of bee pollen obtained from *Cistus ladaniferus* has been shown to have inhibitory effects on bone resorption in femoral tissues and osteoclast-like cell formation in bone marrow cell culture *in vitro* [358]. The femoral-diaphyseal or -metaphyseal tissues of rats were cultured for 48 hours in a medium containing either vehicle, bone-resorbing factor, or bone-resorbing factor plus bee pollen extracts (10, 100, or 1000 μg/ml of medium). Culture with parathyroid hormone (PTH; 10^{-7} M), prostaglandin E_2 (PGE_2; 10^{-5} M), or 1, 25-dihydroxyvitamin D_3 (10^{-6} M) caused a significant decrease in calcium content in the diaphyseal or metaphyseal tissues. These decreases were completely prevented in the presence of bee pollen extracts (10, 100, or 1000 μg/ml) [358]. The presence of PTH caused a significant increase in medium glucose consumption and lactic acid production in the diaphyseal or metaphyseal tissues. These increases were significantly inhibited after culture with bee pollen extracts (10, 100, or 1000 μg/ml) [358].

Mouse bone marrow cells were cultured for 7 days in the presence of bone-resorbing factor *in vitro* [358]. Culture with PTH, PGE_2, tumor necrosis factor-α (TNF- α; 10 ng/ml), or lypopolysaccharide (LPS; 10 μg/ml) caused a significant increase in osteoclast-like cell formation. These increases were significantly inhibited in the presence of bee pollen extracts (10, 50, or 100 μg/ml) [358], indicating that bee pollen extract has been shown to have an inhibitory effect on osteoclastic bone resorption *in vitro*.

Effect of Bee-related Products on Bone

The effects of bee pollen, propolis, and royal jelly extracts on osteogenesis have been compared [359]. The effects of water-solubilized extract or ethanol-solubilized extract obtained from propolis on bone calcium content *in vitro* have been examined [356, 359]. The water-solubilized extract (100 μg/ml of medium) caused a significant increase in bone calcium content. The ethanol-solubilized extract (10, 50, or 100 μg/ml) did not have a significant effect on bone calcium content. Meanwhile, royal jelly (50 or 100 μg/ml) did not have a suppressive effect on PTH-induced increase in osteoclast-like cell formation in bone marrow culture *in vitro* [359]. Thus, among bee-related factors, bee pollen extract has a potential anabolic effect on bone calcification.

Active Components of Bee Pollen Extract

The effects of the fractionated extracts obtained from bee pollen on bone calcium content and osteoclast-like cell formation *in vitro* has been examined [369]. The femoral-diaphyseal and -metaphyseal tissues of rats were cuktured for 48 hours in a medium containing either vehicle or the water-solubilized extract with the menbrane fractions obtained from bee pollen. The active component of bee pollen in increasing calcium content in the diaphyseal tissues was seen in the fraction of molecular weight (MW) of less than 1000, and it was not observed in fractions of greater than MW 1000 [360]. Culture with fractionated bee pollen extract (25 or 50 μg/ml of medium) of less than MW 1000 caused a significant increase in calcium content in the diaphyseal or metaphyseal tissues.

PTH (10^{-6} M)-induced decrease in diaphyseal calcium content was significantly prevented in the presence of the fractionated bee pollen extracts (10 μg/ml) of less than MW 1000 or greater than MW 1000 [360]. Mouse marrow cells were cultured for 7 days in a medium containing PTH in the presence or absence of the fractionated bee pollen extract (10 or 50 μg/ml) [360]. PTH-induced increase in osteoclast-like cell formation was markedly suppressed in the presence of extracts of less than MW 1000 as compared with that in the presence of fractions of greater than MW 1000 [360].

The effects of the fractionated bee pollen extracts of less than MW 1000 in increasing diaphyseal calcium content and in inhibiting PTH-induced osteoclastic cell formation were significantly decreased upon heat treatment for 20 and 60 min at 80 ℃. This observation demonstrates that the active component of bee pollen *Cistus ladaniferus* extract, which stimulates osteoblastic bone formation and inhibits osteoclastic bone resorption, is present in the fraction with MW less than 1000 [360]. This suggests that an identical factor may regulate osteoblastogenesis and osteoclastogenesis.

Intake of Bee Pollen Extract Prevents Bone Loss

Bee pollen extract has stimulatory effects on osteoblastic bone formation and suppressive effects on osteoclastic bone resorption *in vitro*. Whether bee pollen extract has an anabolic effect on bone metabolism *in vivo* has been examined.

Oral administration of the water-solubilized extract obtained from the pollen of *Cistus ladaniferus* to rats caused a significant increase in calcium content in the femoral-diaphyseal and -metaphyseal tissues, indicating that the extract exerts anabolic effects on bone components *in vivo* [356]. It has been speculated that the active component in the water-solubilized extract obtained from the pollen of *Cistus ladaniferus* is transported in the intestine and acts on osteoblatic cells in bone tissues. If the active component is transported in the intestine, it may not be a high molecular-weight compound. The active component in bee pollen extract is found in the fraction of less than MW 1000 [360].

The effect of bee pollen *Cistus ladaniferus* extract on ovariectomy (OVX)-induced bone loss *in vivo* has been examined [361]. The water-solubilized extracts were obtained from the bee pollen of *Cistus ladaniferus*. Cistus extract (50 or 100 mg/kg body weight) was orally administered once daily for 30 days to OVX rats. The analysis using a peripheral quantitative computed tomography showed that OVX-induced a significant decrease in mineral content, mineral density, and polar strength strain index in the femoral-metaphyseal tissues. These decreases were significantly prevented after the administration of cistus extract (100 mg/kg) [361]. Moreover, OVX-induced a significant decrease in calcium content in the femoral-diaphyseal and -metaphyseal tissues. This decrease was significantly prevented after the administration of cistus extract (50 or 100 mg/kg) [361]. This study demonstrates that cistus extract has a preventive effect on OVX-induced bone loss *in vivo*.

The effects of bee pollen cistus extract on serum and bone biochemical components in streptozotocin (STZ)-diabetic rats have been deterimined [362]. The water-solubilized extracts were obtained from the bee pollen of *Cistus ladaniferus*. Rats received a single subcutaneous administration of STZ (60 mg/kg body weight), which induces type I diabetes, and then the animals received the administration of the water-solubilized extract (50, 100, or 200 mg/kg) of bee pollen once daily for 14 days. The administration of STZ caused a significant decrease in body weight and a significant increase in serum glucose, triglyceride and calcium levels, indicating a diabetic state. These alterations were significantly prevented after the administration of the extract (50, 100, or 200 mg/kg) [362]. Serum inorganic phosphorus concentration was significantly decreased in STZ-diabetic rats, and the decrease was significantly prevented after the administration of the extract of 100 or 200 mg/kg [362].

Alkaline phosphatase activity and calcium content in the femoral-diaphyseal and -metaphyseal tissues were significantly decreased in STZ-diabetic rats. These decreases were significantly prevented after the administration of the extract of 100 or 200 mg/kg [362]. The diaphyseal DNA content was also significantly decreased in STZ-diabetic rats. This decrease was significantly prevented after the administration of the extract of 100 or 200 mg/kg [362]. This finding demonstrates that the intake of bee pollen extract has preventive effects on bone loss in STZ-diabetic rats, and that the intake has partial restorative effects on serum biochemical findings with the diabetic state.

Bee pollen is used as nutrient factors in Europe and Japan. Bee pollen extract has shown to have a preventive effect on osteoporosis due to stimulating osteoblastic bone formation and an inhibitory effect on osteoclastic bone resorption. An identification of active component in bee pollen extract remains to be elucidated.

Conclusion

Royal jelly, propolis and bee pollen, which are bee-related products, are generally used as a nutrient factor. Supplemental intake of dietary bee products may help to prevent bone loss with increasing age. Among of royal jelly, propolis and bee pollen, the water-soluble extract obtained from bee pollen *Cistus ladaniferus* has been found to have anabolic effects on bone tissues *in vitro*. Bee pollen extract has stimulatory effects on osteoblastic bone formation and suppressive effects on osteoclastogenesis and bone resorption *in vitro*. Active components are present in less than MW 1000 in bee pollen extract. Supplemental intake of bee pollen extract prevented bone loss in overiectomized and streptozotocin-induced diabetic rats *in vivo*. Supplemental intake of bee pollen extract may play a role in the prevention and treatment of osteoporosis.

Conclusion

Bone loss with aging induces osteoporosis. The decrease in bone mass, which is maintained through osteoblastic cells and osteoclastic cells in bone tissues, leads to bone fracture. Bone loss may be due to decreased osteoblastic bone formation and increased osteoclastic bone resorption with increasing age. Nutritional and functional food factors are needed to prevent bone loss. This may be important in maintaining bone health in long life.

The author has focused on the role of nutritional factors in the prevention and treatment of osteoporosis since year 1984, and it has been firstly demonstrated that zinc, an essential trace element, has stimulatory effects on osteoblastic bone formation and suppressive effects on osteoclastic bone resorption, thereby increasing bone mass. After that, isoflavone (including genistein and daidzein), which are contained in soybean, menaquinone-7, an analogue of vitamin K_2 which is abundant in fermented soybeans, has been demonstrated to stimulate osteoblastic bone formation and to inhibit osteoblastic bone resorption. Moreover, among various carotenoids (including lutein, lycopene, β-carotein, and astaxanthin), β-cryptoxanthin, which is largely in Satuma mandarin (*C. unchiu* MARC), has been found to uniquely have stimulatory effects on osteoblastic bone formation and suppressive effects on osteoblastic bone resorption. Also, flavonoid *p*-hydroxycinnamic acid, which is present in many plant and fruits, has also been shown to have an osteogenic effect on bone, whereas other cinnamic acid-related compounds do not have an effect on bone. These findings were the first time in this field. These factors have been found to regulate gene expression of various proteins that are related to the regulation of osteoblastic and osteoclastic cell functions. This was partly contributed to the clarification of a new molecular mechnism in the regulation of bone homeostasis.

The dietary supplementation of zinc, genistein, menaquinone-7, β-cryptoxanthin and *p*-hydroxycinnamic acid has been shown to have restorative effects on bone loss induced in ovariectomized rats, which are an animal model of osteoporosis, due to stimulating osteoblastic bone formation and suppressing osteoclastic bone resorption. Moreover, supplemental intake of these factors has been demonstrated to have anabolic effects on bone metabolism in humans including postmenopausal women. Food chemical factors play an important role in bone health and osteoporosis prevention with increasing age and various pathophysiologic states.

As introduced in this book, quercetin, curcumin, catechin, and honokiol, which are bio-synthesized in various plants, has also been shown to have stimulatory effects on osteoblastic bone formation and suppressive effects on osteoclastic bone resorption. These factors have been shown to have restorative effects on osteoporosis in animal models. In addition, the bioactive components, which are extracted from other food and plants (including wasabi leafstalk, marine alga *S. horneri*, and bee pollen from *C. ladaniferus*), have been found to have osteogenic effects and preventive effects on osteoprosis. In feature, we may find out other nutritional and food factors, which have benefit effects on the treatment of osteoporosis.

Anti-resorptive agents have long been the preferred standard of care for the amelioration of bone loss, because the processes of bone resorption and bone formation are tightly "coupled", anti-resorptive therapies are also observed clinically to simultaneously suppress bone formation leading to a "low bone turnover state". Although in general anti-resorptive agents do an excellent job of preventing additional bone loss, they do not allow for adequate regeneration of lost bone mass. Drugs, which are used clinically in the treatment of osteoporosis, are mainly based on the action of osteoclastic bone resorption. An intensive effort has begun to identify or develop anabolic agents capable of rebuilding lost bone mineral density. At present teriparatide, a fragment of human parathyroid hormone is only the United State Food and Drug Administration (FDA) approved anabolic agent currently available. This agent represents a significant leap forward but as a biologic based agent its use is limited by high cost and the need for daily injection. Furthermore, therapy is not recommended for more than 2 years due to the potential for osteosarcoma. As a consequence, there is intense interest in the identification of additional anabolic agents.

Clinical compounds that stimulate bone formation are under development. As described in this book, various chemical factors, which stimulate bone formation, are found in various food and plants. These factors may be useful in the therapy of osteoporosis. It has been expected that studies of the chemical structure-related activity of biofactors from food and plants will lead to the development of new drugs that stimulate bone formation and inhibit bone resorption. Analogues, which are synthesized with origination of bioactive chemicals derived from food factors, may be developed as novel drugs that reveal potent-osteogenic effects for the treatment of osteolysis which is induced in various diseases including osteoporosis, inflammation, obesity, diabetes, cancer cell bone metastasis, and bone fracture.

Interestingly, the osteogenic effects of vitamin D_3, vitamin K_2 (menaquinone-7), and genistein have been demonstrated to be synergistically enhanced with the combination of zinc. These ingredients may have potential effects in the prevention and treatment of osteoporosis as a supplemental drug.

The functional food factors will be expected as new biomedical treatment for osteoporosis.

References

[1] Riggs B L, Jowsey J, Kelly PJ, Jones JD, Maher FT (1969) Effect of sex hormones on bone in primary osteoporosis. *J Clin Invest* 48: 1065-1072.

[2] Cooper C, Melton J III (1995) Epidemiology of osteoporosis. *Trends Endocrinol Metab* 3: 224-229.

[3] Weitzmann MN, Pacifici R (2006) Estrogen deficiency and bone loss: an inflammatory tale. *J Clin Invest* 116: 1186-1194.

[4] Bonjour J-P, Schurch M-A, Rizzori R (1996) Nutritional aspects of hip fracture. *Bone* 18: 1395-1445.

[5] Yamaguchi M (2010) *Nutritional Factors and Osteoporosis Prevention*. New York, Nova Science Publishers, Inc.

[6] Manolagas SC (2000) Birth and death of bone cells: basic regulatory mechanisms and implications for the pathogenesis and treatment of osteoporosis. Endcr Rev 21:115-137.

[7] Baron R, Vignery A, Horowitz M (1984) Lymphocytes, macrophages and the regulation of bone remodeling. *Bone Miner Res* 2:175-243.

[8] Zaidi M, Blair HC, Moonga BS, Abe E, Huang C L-H (2003) Osteoclastogenesis, bone resorption, and osteoblast-based therapeutics. *J Bone Miner Res* 18: 599-609.

[9] Chambers TJ, Fuller K (2011) How are osteoclasts induced to resorb bone? *Ann N Y Acad Sci* 1240:1-6.

[10] Raggatt LJ, Partridge NC (2010) Cellular and molecular mechanisms of bone modeling. *J Biol Chem* 285:25103-25108.

[11] Canalis E, McCarthy T, Centrella M (1988) Growth factors and the regulation of bone remodeling. *J Clin Invest* 81: 277-281.

[12] Chen G, Deng C, Li YP (2012) TGF-β and BMP signaling in osteoblast differentiation and bone formation. *Int J Biol Sci* 8:272-288.

[13] Inoue K, Matsuda K, Itoh M, Kawaguchi H, Tomoike H, Aoyagi T, Nagai R, Hori M, Nakamura Y, Tanaka T (2002) Osteopenia and male-specific sudden cardiac death in mice lacking a zinc transporter gene, Znt5. *Hum Mol Genet* 15:1775-1784.

[14] Khadeer MA, Sahu SN, Bai G, Abdulla S, Gupta A (2005) Expression of the zinc transporter ZIP1 in osteoclasts. *Bone,* 37:296-304.

[15] Nakashima K, Zhou X, Kunkel G, Zhang Z, Deng JM, Behringer RR, de Crombrugghe B (2002) The novel zinc finger-containing transcription factor osterix is required for osteoblast differentiation and bone formation. *Cell* 108:17-29.

[16] Shen ZJ, Nakamoto T, Tsuji K, Nifuji A, Miyazono K, Komori T, Hirai H, Noda M (2002) Negative regulation of bone morphogenetic protein/Smad signaling by Cas-interacting zinc finger protein in osteoblasts. *J Biol Chem,* 277: 29840-29846.

[17] Jones DC, Wein MN, Oukka M, Hofstaetter JG, Glimcher MJ, Glimcher LH (2006) Schnur regulation of adult bone mass by the zinc finger adapter protein ri-3. *Science* 312: 1223-1227.

[18] Shin JN, Kim I, Lee JS, Koh GY, Lee ZH, Kim HH (2002) A novel zinc finger protein that inhibits osteoclastogenesis and the function of tumor necrosis factor receptor-associated factor 6. *J Biol Chem,* 277:8346-53.

[19] Melton LJ 3rd, Chrischilles EA, Cooper C, Lane AW, Riggs BL (1992) Perspective. How many women have osteoporosis? *J Bone Miner Res* 7:1005-1010.

[20] Leslie WD, Rubin MR, Schwartz AV, Kanis JA (2012) Type 2 diabetes and bone. *J Bone Miner Res* 27:2231-2237.

[21] Blanchard JF, Ludwig S, Wajda A, Dean H, Anderson K, Kendall O, Depew N (1996) Incidence and prevalence of diabetes in Manitoba, 1986-1991. *Diabetes Care* 19:807-811.

[22] Wild S, Roglic G, Green A, Sicree R, King H (2004) Global prevalence of diabetes: estimates for the year 2000 and projections for 2030, *Diabetes Care* 27:104753.

[23] Nielson CM, Srikanth P, Orwoll ES (2012) Obesity and fracture in men and women: An epidemiologic perspective. *J Bone Miner Res* 27:1-10.

[24] Bilezikian JP, Davidson M, Hendrix S, Liu L, Louie M (2005). Co-morbidity of decreased bone mineral density (BMD) and increased cholesterol levels among women aged 65 years and older: results from NHANES III. *ASBMR 27th Annu Meet.* SU130.

[25] Cui LH, Shin MH, Chung EK, Lee YH, Kweon SS, Park KS, Choi JS (2005) Association between bone mineral densities and serum lipid profiles of pre- and post-menopausal rual women in South Korea. *Osteoporos Int* 16:1975-1981.

[26] Parhami F, Tintut Y, Beamer WG, Gharavi N, Goodman W, Demer LL (2001) Atherogenic high-fat diet reduces bone mineralization in mice. *J Bone Miner Res* 16:182-188.

[27] Pirih F, Lu J, Ye F, Bezouglaia O, Atti E, Ascenzi M-G, Tetradis S, Demer L, Aghaloo T, Tintut Y (2012) Adverse effects of hyperlipidemia on bone regeneration and strength. *J Bone Miner Res* 27:309-318.

[28] Prasad AS, Halsted JA, Nadimi M (1961) Syndrome of iron deficiency anemia, hepatosplenomegaly, hupogonadism, dwarfism and geophagia. *Am J Med* 31:532-546.

[29] Burch RE, Hahn HK, Sullivan JF (1975) Newer aspects of the roles of zinc, manganese, and copper in human nutrition. *Clin Chem* 21:501-520.

[30] Parisi AF, Vallee BL (1969) Zinc metalloenzyme: Characteristic and significance in biology and medicine. *Am J Clin Nutr* 22:1222-1230.

[31] Hsieh HS, Navia JM (1980) Zinc deficiency and bone formation in guinea pig alveolar implants. *J Nutr* 110:1581-1588.

[32] Oner G, Bhaumick B, Bala RM (1984) Effect of zinc deficiency on serum somatomedin levels and skeletal growth in young rats. *Endocrinology* 114:1860-1863.

[33] Hurley LS (1981) Tetratogenic aspects of manganese, zinc, and copper nutrition. *Physiological Reviews* 61:249-295.

[34] da Cunha Ferreira RM, Marguiegui IM, Elizaga IV (1989) Tetratogenicity of zinc deficiency in the rat: Study of the fetal skeleton. *Tetratology* 39:181-194.

[35] Leek JC, Vogler JB, Gershwin ME, Golub MS, Hurley LS, Hendrickx AG (1984) Studies of marginal zinc deprivation in rhesus monkeys. V. Fetal and infant skeletal defects. *Am J Clin Nutr* 40:1203-1212.

[36] Ronaghy HA, Reinhold JG, Mahloudji M, Ghavami P, Spirey Fox MR, Halstead JA (1984) Zinc supplementation of malnourished schoolboys in Iran: Increased growth and other effects. *Am J Clin Nutr* 40:1203-1212.

[37] Haumont S (1961) Distribution of zinc in bone tissues. *J Histochem Cytochem* 9:141.

[38] Hurley LS, Shyy-Hwa T (1972) Alleviation of tetratogenic effects of zinc deficiency by simultaneous lack of calcium. *Am J Phys* 222:322-325.

[39] Masters DG, Keen CL, Lonnerdal B, Hurley LS (1986) Release of zinc from maternal tissues during zinc deficiency or simultaneous zinc and calcium deficiency in the pregnant rat. *J Nutr* 116:2148-2154.

[40] Murray EJ, Messer HH (1981) Turnover of bone zinc during normal and accelerated bone loss in rats. *J Nutr* 111:1641-1647.

[41] Sherman SS, Smith JC, Tobin JD, Soares JH (1989) Ovariectomy, dietary zinc, and bone metabolism in retired breeder rats. *Am J Clin Nutr* 49:1184-1191.

[42] Aitken JM (1976) Factors affecting the distribution of zinc in the human skeleton. *Calcif Tissue Res* 20:23-30.

[43] Sauer GR, Wuthier RE (1990) Distribution of zinc in the avian growth plate. *J Bone Mineral Res* 5 (Suppl. 2):S162.

[44] Lappalainer R, Knuuttila M, Lammi S, Alhava EM (1983) Fluoride content related to the elemental composition, mineral density and strength of bone in healthy and chronically diseased persons. *J Chronic Disease* 36:707-713.

[45] Reginster JY, Strause LG, Saltman O, Franchimont P (1988) Trace elements and postmenopausal osteoporosis: A preliminary study of decreased serum manganese. *Med Sci Res* 16:337-338.

[46] Herzberg M, Foldes J, Steinberg R, Menczel J (1990) Zinc excretion in osteoporotic women. *J Bone Mineral Res* 5:251-257.

[47] Yamaguchi M, Takahashi K (1984) Role of zinc as an acivator of bone metabolism in weanling rats. *Jpn J Bone Metab* 2:186-191.

[48] Parfitt AM (1990) Bone-forming cells in clinical conditions. In: Hall BK (editor), *Bone Volume 1 The Osteoblast and Osteocyte,* p.351-429, Boca Raton, Florida: Telford Press and CRC Press.

[49] Canalis E, McCarthy T, Centrella M (1988) Growth factors and the regulation of bone remodeling. *J Clin Invest* 81:277-281.

[50] Yamaguchi M, Inamoto K, Suketa Y (1986) Effect of essential trace metals on bone metabolism in weanling rats: Comparison with zinc and other metals` actions. *Res Exp Med* 186:337-342.

[51] Yamaguchi M, Uchiyama M (1987) Preventive effect of zinc for toxic actions of germanium and selenium on bone metabolism in weanling rats. *Res Exp Med* 187:395-400.

[52] Lai YL, Yamaguchi M (2005) Effects of copper on bone component in the femoral tissues of rats: Anabolic effect of zinc is weakened by copper. *Biol Pharm Bull* 28:2296-2301.

[53] Yamaguchi M, Osishi H, Suketa Y (1987) Stimulatory effect of zinc on bone formation in tissue culture. *Biochem Pharmacol* 36:4007-4012.

[54] Yamaguchi M, Oishi H, Suketa Y (1988) Zinc stimulation of bone protein synthesis in tissue culture. Activation of aminoacyl-tRNA synthetase. *Biochem Pharmacol* 37:4075-4080.

[55] Yamaguchi M, Matsui R (1989) Effect of dipicolinate, a chelator of zinc, on bone protein synthesis in tissue culture. The essential role of zinc. *Biochem Pharmacol* 38:4485-4489.

[56] Shimokawa N, Yamaguchi M (1992) Characterization of bone protein components with polyacrylamide gel electrophoresis: Effects of zinc and hormones in tissue culture. *Mol Cell Biochem* 117:153-158.

[57] Yamaguchi M, Sakashita T (1986) Enhancement of vitamin D_3 effect on bone metabolism in weanling rats orally administered zinc sulphate. *Acta Endocrinol* 111:285-288.

[58] Yamaguchi M, Yamaguchi R (1986) Action of zinc on bone metabolism in rats. Increase in alkaline phosphatase activity and DNA content. *Biochem Pharmacol* 35:773-777.

[59] Yamaguchi M, Inamoto K (1986) Differential effects of calcium-regulating hormones on bone metabolismin weanling rats orally administered zinc sulfate. *Metabolism* 35:1044-1047.

[60] McDonnell DP, Mongelsdorf DJ, Pike JW, Haussler MR, O'Malley BW (1987) Molecular cloning of complementary DNA encoding the avian receptor for vitamin D. *Science* 235:1214-1217.

[61] Yamaguchi M, Oishi H (1989) Effect of 1,25-dihydroxyvitamin D_3 on bone metabolism in tissue culture. Enhancement of this steroid effect by zinc. *Biochem Pharmacol* 38:3453-3459.

[62] Yamaguchi M, Kitajima T (1991) Effect of estrogen on bone metabolism in tissue culture: Enhancement of the steroid effect by zinc. *Res Exp Med* 191:145-154.

[63] Lutz W, Burritt MF, Nixon DE, Kao PC, Kumar R (2000) Zinc increases the activity of vitamin D-dependent promoters in osteoblasts. *Biochem Biophys Res Commun* 271: 1-7.

[64] Hashizume M, Yamaguchi M (1993) Stimulatory effect of β-alanyl-L-histidinato zinc on cell proliferation is dependent on protein synthesis in osteoblastic MC3T3-E1 cells. *Mol Cell Biochem* 122:59-64.

[65] Hashizume M, Yamaguchi M (1994) Effect of β-alanyl-L-histidinato zinc on differentiation of osteoblastic MC3T3-E1 cells: Increases in alkaline phosphatase activity and protein concentration. *Mol Cell Biochem* 131:19-24.

[66] Yamaguchi M, Hashizume M (1994) Effect of β-alanyl-L-histidinato zinc on proein components in osteoblastic MC3T3-E1 cells: Increases in osteocalcin, insulin-like growth factor-I and transforming growth factor-β. *Mol Cell Biochem* 136:163-169.

[67] Matsui T, Yamaguchi M (1995) Zinc modulation of insulin-like growth factor's effect in osteoblastic MC3T3-E1 cells. *Peptides* 16:1063-1068.

[68] Yamaguchi M, Fukagawa M (2005) Role of zinc in regulation of protein tyrosine phosphatase activity in osteoblastic MC3T3-E1 cells: Zinc modulation of insulin-like growth factor-I's effect. *Calcif Tissue Int* 76:32-38.

[69] Yamaguchi M, Kishi S, Hashizume M (1994) Effect of zinc-chelating dipeptides on osteoblastic MC3T3-E1 cells: Activation of aminoacyl-tRNA synthetase. *Peptides* 15:1367-1371.

[70] Yamaguchi M, Matsui T (1996) Stimulatory effect of zinc-chelating dipeptide on deoxyribonucleic acid synthesis in osteoblastic MC3T3-E1 cells. *Peptide* 17:1207-1211.

[71] Yamaguchi M, Goto M, Uchiyama S, Nakagawa T (2008) Effect of zinc on gene expression in osteoblastic MC3T3-E1 cells: enhancement of Runx2, OPG, and regucalcin mRNA expressions. *Mol Cell Biochem,* 312:157-66.

[72] Yamaguchi M, Segawa Y, Shimokawa N, Tsuzuike N, Tagashira E (1992) Inhibitory effect of β-alanyl-L-histidinato zinc on bone resorption in tissue culture. *Pharmacology* 45:292-300.

[73] Yamaguchi M, Hashizume M (1994) Effect of parathyroid hormone and interleukin-1α in osteoblastic MC3T3-E1 cells: Interaction with β-alanyl-L-histidinato zinc. *Peptides* 15:633-636.

[74] Kishi S, Yamaguchi M (1994) Inhibitory effect of zinc compounds on osteoclast-like cell formation in mouse marrow cultures. *Biochem Pharmacol* 48:1225-1230.

[75] Yamaguchi M, Kishi S (1996) Zinc compounds inhibit osteoclast-like cell formation at the earlier stage of rat marrow culture but not osteoclast function. *Mol Cell Biochem* 158:171-177.

[76] Yamaguchi M, Kishi S (1995) Inhibitory effect of zinc-chelating dipeptide on parathyroid hormone-stimulated osteoclast-like cell formation in mouse marrow cultures: Involvement of calcium signaling. *Peptides* 16:629-633.

[77] Tanaka S, Nakamura I, Inoue J, Oda H, Nakamura K (2003) Osteoclastogenesis, bone resorption, and osteoclast-based therapeutics. *J. Bone Miner. Res.*, 18: 599-609.

[78] Asagiri M, Takayanagi H (2007) The molecular understanding of osteoclast differentiation. *Bone* 40:251-264.

[79] Anderson DM, Marashovsky E, Billingoley WL, Dougall WC, Tometsko ME, Roux ER, Teepe MC, DuBose RF, Cosman D, Galibert L (1997) A homologue of the TNF receptor and its ligand enhances T-cell growth an dentritic-cell function. *Nature* (London) 390:175-179.

[80] Yasuda H, Shima N, Nakagawa N, Yamaguchi K, Kinosaki M, Mochizuki S, Tomoyasu A, Yano K, Goto M, Murakami A, Tsuda E, Morinaga T, Higashio K, Udagawa N, Takahashi N, Suda T (1998) Osteoclast differentiation factor is a ligand for osteoprotegerin/osteoclastogenesis-inhibitory factor and is identical to TRANCE/RANKL. *Proc Natl Acad Sci USA* 95:3597-3602.

[81] Tsuda E, Goto M, Mochizuki S, Yano K, Kobayashi F, Morinaga T, Higashio K (1997) Isolation of a novel cytokine from human fibroblasts that specifically inhibits osteoclastogenesis. *Biochem Biophys Res Commun* 234:137-142.

[82] Inoue J, Ishida T, Tsukamoto N, Kobayashi N, Naito A, Azuma S, Yamamoto T (2000) Tumor necrosis factor receptor-associated factor (TRAF) family: adaptor proteins that mediate cytokine signaling. *Exp Cell Res* 254:14-24.

[83] Yamaguchi M, Uchiyma S (2004) Receptor activator of Nf-κB ligand (RANKL)-stimulated osteoclastogenesis in mouse marrow culture is suppressed by zinc in vitro. *Int J Mol Med* 14:81-85.

[84] Zou W, Hikim I, Tschoep K, Endres S, Zvi B-S (2001) Tumor necrosis factor-mediated RANK ligand stimulation of osteoclast differentiation by an autocrine mechanism. *J Cell Biochem* 83:70-83.

[85] Ma ZJ, Yamaguchi M (2000) Alteration in bone components with increasing age of newborn rats: role of zinc in bone growth. *J Bone Miner Metab* 18:264-270.

[86] Ma ZJ, Yamaguchi M (2001) Role of endogenous zinc in the enhancement of bone protein synthesis associated with bone growth of newborn rats. *J Bone Miner Metab* 19:38-44.

[87] Ma ZJ, Misawa H, Yamaguchi M (2001) Stimulatory effect of zinc on insulin-like growth factor-I and transforming growth factor-β1 production with bone growth of newborn rats. *Int J Mol Med* 8:623-628.

[88] Gabbitas B, Pash J, Canalis E (1994) Regulation of insulin-like groth factor-II synthesis in bone cell cultures by skeletal growth factors. *Endocrinology* 135:284-289.

[89] Asahina I, Sampath TK, Nishimura I, Hauschka PV (1999) Human osteogenic protein-1 induces both chondroblastic and osteoblastic differentiation of osteoprogenitor cells derived from newborn rat calvaria. *J Cell Biol* 123:921-933.

[90] Ma ZJ and Yamaguchi M (2001) Stimulatory effect of zinc and growth factor on bone protein component in newborn rats: Enhancement with zinc and insulin-like growth factor-I. *Int J Mol Med* 7:73-78.

[91] Ma ZJ, Yamaguchi M (2001) Stimulatory effect of zinc on deoxyribonucleic acid synthesis in bone growth of newborn rats: Enhancement with zinc and insulin-like growth factor-I. *Calcif Tissue Int* 69:158-163.

[92] Barnes GL, Kostenuik PJ, Gerstenfeld LC, Eihorn TA (1999) Growth factor regulation of fracture repair. *J Bone Miner Res* 14:1805-1815.

[93] Eihorn TA (1998) The cell and molecular biology of fracture healing. *Clin Orthop* 355S:S7-S21.

[94] Bolander ME (1998) Regulation of fracture repair by growth factors. *Proc Soc Exp Biol Med* 200:165-170.

[95] Igarashi A, Yamaguchi M (1999) Increase in bone protein components with healing rat fractures: Enhancement by zinc treatment. *Int J Mol Med* 4:615-620.

[96] Igarashi A, Yamaguchi M (2001) Increase in bone growth factors with healing rat fractures: The enhancing effect of zinc. *Int J Mol Med* 8:433-438.

[97] Igarashi A, Yamaguchi M (2002) Characterization of the increase in bone 66 kDa protein component with healing rat fractures: Stimulatory effect of zinc. *Int J Mol Med* 9:503-508.

[98] Igarashi A, Yamaguchi M (2003) Great increase in bone 66 kDa protein and osteocalcin at later stage with healing rat fractures: Effect of zinc treament. *Int J Mol Med* 11:223-228.

[99] Yamaguchi M, Igarashi A, Misawa H, Tsurusaki Y (2003) Enhancement of albumin expression in bone tissues with healing rat fractures. *J Cell Biochem* 89:356-363.

[100] Ishida K, Sawada N, Yamaguchi M (2004) Expression of albumin in bone tissues and osteoblastic cells: Involvement of hormone regulation. *Int J Mol Med* 14:891-895.

[101] Ishida K, Yamaguchi M (2004) Role of albumin in ostoblastic cells: Enhancement of cell proliferation and suppression of alkaline phosphatase activity. *Int J Mol Med* 14:1077-1081.

[102] Ishida K, Yamaguchi M (2005) Albumin regulates Runx2 and α1 (I) collagen mRNA expression in osteoblastic cells: Comparison with insulin-like growth factor-I. *Int J Mol Med* 16:689-694.

[103] Igarashi A, Yamaguchi M (1999) Stimulatory effect of zinc acexamate administration on fracture healing of the femoral-diaphyseal tissues in rats. *Gen Pharmacol* 32:463-469.

[104] Yamaguchi M, Ozaki K (1990) A new zinc compound, β-alanyl-L-histidinato zinc, stimulates bone growth in weanling rats. *Res Exp Med* 190:105-110.

[105] Yamaguchi M, Miwa H (1991) Stimulatory effect of beta-alanyl-L-histidinato zinc on bone formation in tissue culture. *Pharmacology* 42:230-240.

[106] Samuchson J (1967) Mechanism for the exchange of the calcium in bone mineral. *Nature* 216:193-194.

[107] Yamaguchi M, Ohtaki J (1991) Effect of beta-alanyl-L-histidinato zinc on osteoblastic MC3T3-E1 cells: Increases in alkaline phosphatase and proliferation. *Pharmacology* 43:225-232.

[108] Yamaguchi M, Kishi S (1994) Effect of zinc-chelating dipeptide on bone metabolism in weanling rats: Comparison with β-alanyl-L-histidinato zinc-related compounds. *Peptides* 15:671-673.

[109] Yamaguchi M, Kishi S (1994) Comparison of the effect of β-alanyl-L-histidinato zinc and its zinc-chelating ligand on bone metabolism in tissue culture. *Biol Pharm Bull* 17:522-526.

[110] Yamaguchi M, Ozaki K, Suketa Y (1989) Alteration in bone metabolism with increasing age: Effects of zinc and vitamin D_3 in aged rats. *J Pharmacobio-Dyn* 12:67-73.

[111] Yamaguchi M, Ozaki K (1990) Aging affects cellular zinc and protein synthesis in the femoral diaphysis of rats. *Res Exp Med* 190:295-300.

[112] Yamaguchi M, Ozaki K (1990) Effect of the new zinc compound beta-alanyl-L-histidinato zinc on bone metabolism in elderly rats. *Pharmacology* 41:345-349.

[113] Kishi S, Yamaguchi M (1994) Stimulatory effect of β-alanyl-L-histidinato zinc on alkaline phosphatase activity in bone tissue from elderly rats: Comparison with zinc sulfate action. *Biol Pharm Bull* 17:345-347.

[114] Yamaguchi M, Ehara Y (1995) Zinc decrease and bone metabolism in the femoral-metaphyseal tissues of rats with skeletal unloading. *Calcif Tissue Int* 57:218-223.

[115] Yamaguchi M, Ehara Y (1996) Effect of essential trace metal on bone metabolism in the femoral-metaphyseal tissues of rats with skeletal unloading: Comparison with zinc-chelating dipeptide. *Calcif Tissue Int* 59:27-32.

[116] Morey ER, Baylink DJ (1978) Inhibition of bone formation during spaceflight. *Science* 201:1138-1141.

[117] Yamaguchi M, Ozaki K, Hoshi T (1990) β-Alanyl-L-histidinato zinc prevents skeletal unloading-induced disorder of bone metabolism in rats. *Res Exp Med* 190:289-294.

[118] Maloney NA, Ott SM, Alfrey AC, Miller NL, Coburn JW, Sherrard DJ (1982) Histological quantitation of aluminium in iliac from patients with renal failure. *J Lab Clin Med* 99:206-216.

[119] Yamaguchi M, Ozaki K (1990) Beta-alanyl-L-histidinato zinc prevents the toxic effect of aluminium on bone metabolism in weanling rats. *Pharmacology* 41:338-344.

[120] Segawa Y, Tsuzuike N, Tagashira E, Yamaguchi M (1992) Preventive effect of β-alanyl-L-histidinato zinc on bone metabolism in rats fed on low-calcium and vitamin D-deficient diets. *Res Exp Med* 192:213-219.

[121] Segawa Y, Tsuzuike N, Itokazu Y, Tagashira E, Yamaguchi M (1993) Effect of β-alanyl-L-histidinato zinc on bone metabolism in rats with adjuvant arthritis. *Biol Pharm Bull* 16:656-659.

[122] Sugiyama T, Tanaka H, Kawai S (2000) Improvement of periarticular osteoporosis in postmenopausal women with rheumatoid arthritis by beta-alanyl-L-histidinato zinc: a pilot study. *J Bone Miner Metab* 18: 335-338.

[123] Pock WA (1984) The effects of glucocorticoids on bone cell metabolism and function. *Adv Exp Med Biol* 171:111-119.

[124] Segawa Y, Tsuzuike N, Itokazu Y, Tagashira E, Yamaguchi M (1992) β-Alanyl-L-histidinato zinc prevents hydrocortisone-induced disorder of bone metabolism in rats. *Res Exp Med* 192:317-322.

[125] Johnston CC Jr, Hui SL, Witt RM, Appledonn R, Baker RS, Longcope C (1985) Early menopausal changes in bone mass and sex steroids. *J Clin Endocrinol Metab* 61:905-911.

[126] Goulding A, Gold E (1987) Effects of chronic prednisolone treatment on bone resorption and bone composition in intact and ovariectomized rats receiving β-estradiol. *Endocrinology* 122:482-487.

[127] Segawa Y, Tsuzuike N, Tagashira E, Yamaguchi M (1993) Preventive effect of β-alanyl-L-histidinato zinc on the deterioration of bone metabolism in ovariectomized rats. *Biol Pharm Bull* 16:486-489.

[128] Yamaguchi M, Kishi S (1993) Prolonged administration of β-alanyl-L-histidinato zinc prevents bone loss in ovariectomized rats. *Jap J Pharmacol* 63:203-207.

[129] Kishi S, Segawa Y, Yamaguchi M (1994) Histomorphological confirmation of the preventive effect of β-alanyl-L-histidinato zinc on bone loss in ovariectomized rats. *Biol Pharm Bull* 17:862-865.

[130] Yamaguchi M, Gao YH (1998) Potent effect of zinc acexamate on bone components in the femoral-metaphyseal tissues of elderly female rats. *Gen Pharmacol* 30:423-427.

[131] Hui SL, Epstein S, Johanston CC (1985) A prospective study of bone mass in patients with type I diabetes. *J Clin Endocrinol Metab* 60:74-80.

[132] Mcnair P (1988) Bone mineral metabolism in human type I diabetes mellitus. *Dan Med Bull* 35:109-121.

[133] Yamaguchi M, Uchiyama S (2003) Preventive effect of zinc acexamate administration in streptozotocin-diabetic rats: Restoration of bone loss. *Int J Mol Med* 12:755-761.

[134] Uchiyama S, Yamaguchi M (2003) Alteration in serum and bone component findings induced in streptozotocin-diabetic rats is restored by zinc acexamate. *Int J Mol Med* 12:949-954.

[135] Relea P, Revilla M, Ripoll E, Arribas I, Villa LF, Rico H (1995) Zinc, biochemical markers of nutrition, and type I osteoporosis. *Age Ageing,* 24: 303-307.

[136] Gur A, Colpan L, Cevik R, Nas K, Jale Sarac A (2005) Comparison of zinc excretion and biochemical markers of bone remodelling in the assessment of the effects of alendronate and calcitonin on bone in postmenopausal osteoporosis. *Clin Biochem* 38: 66-72.

[137] Hill T, Meunier N, Andriollo-Sanchez M, Ciarapica D, Hininger-Favier I, Poloto A, O'Connor JM, Coudray C, Cashman KD (2005) The relationship between the zinc nutritive status and biochemical markers of bone turnover in older European adults: the ZENITH study. *Eur L Clin Nutr* 59 (Suppl 2): S73-S78.

[138] Hyun TH, Barrett-Connor E, Milne DB (2004) Zinc intakes and plasma concentrations in men with osteoporosis: the Rancho Bermardo Study. *Am J Clin Nutr* 80: 715-721.

[139] Rodondi A, Ammann P, Ghilardi-Beuret S, Rizzoli R (2009) Zinc increases the effects of essential amino acids-whey protein supplements in frail elderly. *J Nutr Health Aging* 13: 491-497.

[140] Yamaguchi M, Igarashi A, Sakai M, Degawa H, Ozawa Y (2005) Prolonged intake of dietary fermented isoflavone-rich soybean reinforced with zinc affects circulating bone biochemical markers in aged individuals. *J. Health Sci.*, 51: 191-196.

[141] Yamaguchi M (1995) β-Alanyl-L-histidinato zinc: A potent activator in bone formation. *Curr Med Chem* 1:356-365.

[142] Yamaguchi M (1995) β-Alanyl-L-histidinato zinc and bone resorption. *Gen Pharmac* 26:1179-1183.

[143] Yamaguchi M (1998) Role of zinc in bone formation and bone resorption. *J Trace Elem Exp Med* 11:119-135.

[144] Yamaguchi M (2010) Role of nutritional zinc in the prevention of osteoporosis. *Mol Cell Biochem* 338:241-254.

[145] Yamaguchi M, Igarashi A, Uchiyama S (2004) Bioavailability of zinc yeast in rats: Stimulatory effect on bone calcification in vivo. *J Health Sci* 50:75-81.

[146] Liu Y, Bhalla K, Hill C, Priest DG (1994) Evidence for involvement of tyrosine phosphorylation in taxol-induced apoptosis in a human ovarian tumor cell line. *Biochem Pharmacol* 48: 1265-1272.

[147] Yamaguchi M, Gao YH (1997) Anabolic effect of genistein on bone metabolism in the femoral-metaphyseal tissues of elderly rats is inhibited by the anti-estrogen tamoxifen. *Res Exp Med* 197: 101-107.

[148] Yamaguchi M, Gao YH (1998) Anabolic effect of genistein and genistein on bone metabolism in the femoral-metaphyseal tissues of elderly rats: The genistein effect is enhanced by zinc. *Mol Cell Biochem* 178: 377-382.

[149] Kuiper GG, Lemmen JG, Carlsson B, Corton JC, Safe SH, van der Saag PT, van der Burg B, Gustafsson JA (1998) Interaction of estrogenic chemicals and phytoestrogens with estrogen receptor beta. *Endocrinology* 139: 4252-4263.

[150] Gao YH, Yamaguchi M (1999) Anabolic effect of daizein on cortical bone in tissue culture: Comparison with genistein effect. *Mol Cell Biochem* 194: 93-98.

[151] Yamaguchi M, Zhong JM, Fushimi T (2002) Anabolic effect of phosphogenistein and phosphodaidzein on bone components in rat femoral-metaphyseal tissues in vitro. *J Bone Miner Metab* 20: 148-155.

[152] Yamaguchi M, Ma ZJ (2001) Effect of polyphenols on calcium content and alkaline phosphatase activity in rat femoral tissues *in vitro*. *Biol Pharm Bull* 24: 1437-1430.

[153] Sugimoto E, Yamaguchi M (2000) Anabolic effect of genistein is osteoblastic MC3T3-E1 cells. *Int J Mol Med* 5: 515-520.

[154] Sugimoto E, Yamaguchi M (2000) Stimulatory effect of daidzein in osteoblastic MC3T3-E1 cells. *Biochem Pharmacol* 59: 471-475.

[155] Yamaguchi M, Sugimoto E (2000) Stimulatory effect of genistein and daizein on protein synthesis in osteoblastic MC3T3-E1 cells: Activation of aminoacyl-tRNA synthetase. *Mol Cell Biochem* 214: 97-102.

[156] Yamaguchi M, Weitzmann MN (2009) The estrogen 17β-estradiol and phytoestrogen genistein mediate differential effects on osteoblastic NF-κB activity. *Int J Mol Med* 23: 297-301.

[157] Uchiyama S, Yamaguchi M (2007) Genistein and zinc synergistically enhance gene expression and mineralization in osteoblastic MC3T3-E1 cells. *Int J Mol Med* 19: 213-220.

[158] Majeska RJ, Wuthier RE (1975) Studies on matrix vesicles isolated from chick epiphyseal cartilage. Association of pyrophosphatase and ATPase activities with alkaline phosphatase. *Biochim Biophys Acta* 391: 51-60.

[159] Lian JB, Stein GS, Cannalis E, Roky PG, Boskey AL (1999) Bone formation: Osteoblast lineage cells, growth factor, matrix protein, and the mineralization process. In: Favus MJ (editor), *Primer on the Metabolic Bone Disease and Disorders of Mineral Metabolism,* 4th edition, pp14-29, New York, Lippincott Williams & Wilkins Press.

[160] Pan W, Quarles LD, Song LH, Yu YH, Jiao C, Tang HB, Jiang CH, Deng HW, Li YJ, Zhou HH, Xiao ZS (2005) Genistein stimulates the osteoblastic differentiation via N0/cGMP in bone marrow culture. *J Cell Biochem* 94:307-316.

[161] Tang X, Zhu X, Liu S, Wang S, Ni X (2011) Isoflavones suppress cyclic adenosine 3', 5'-monophosphate regulatory element-mediated trnscription in osteoblastic cell line. *J Nutr Biochem* 22:865-873.

[162] Klein-Nulend J, Fall PM, Raisz LG (1990) Comparison of the effects of synthetic human parathyroid hormone (PTH)-(1-34)-related peptide of malignancy and bovine PTH-(1-34) on bone formation and resorption in organ culture. *Endocrinology* 126: 223-227.

[163] Graves L III, Jilka R L (1990) Comparison of bone and parathyroid hormone as stimulators of osteoclast development and activity in calvarial cell cultures from normal and osteopetrotic (mi/mi) mice. *J Cell Physiol* 145: 102-109.

[164] Klein DC, Raisz LG (1970) Stimulation of bone resorption in tissue culture. *Endocrinology* 86: 1436-1440.

[165] Yamaguchi M, Gao YH (1998) Inhibitory effect of genistein on bone resorption in tissue culture. *Biochem Pharmacol* 55:71-76.

[166] Takahashi N, Yamana H, Yoshiki S, Roodman GD, Mundy GR, Jones SJ, Boyde A, Suda T (1988). Osteoclast-like cell formation and its regulation by osteotropic hormones in mouse bone marrow cultures. *Endocrinology* 122: 1373-1382.

[167] Gao YH, Yamaguchi M (1999) Inhibitory effect of genistein on osteoclast-like cell formation in mouse marrow cultures. *Biochem Pharmacol* 58: 767-772.

[168] Chen XW, Garner SC, Anderson JJ (2002) Isoflavones regulate interleukin-6 and osteoprotegerin synthesis duering osteoblast cell differentiation via an estrogen-receptor-dependent pathway. *Biochem Biophys Res Commun* 295:417-422.

[169] Viereck V, Grundker C, Blaschke S, Siggelkow H, Emons G, Hofbauer LC (2002) Phytoestrogen genistein stimulates the production of osteoprotegerin in human trabecular osteoblasts. *J Cell Biochem* 84:725-735.

[170] Kanatani M, Sugimoto T, Takahashi Y, Kaji H, Kitazawa R, Chihara K (1998) Estrogen via the estrogen receptor blocks cAMP-mediated parathyroid hormon (PTH)-stimulated osteoclast formation. *J Bone Miner Res* 13:854-862.

[171] Garcia Palacios V, Robinson LJ, Borysenko CW, Lehmann T, Kalla SE, Blair HC (2005) Negative regulation of RANKL-induced osteoclastic differentiation in RAW264.7 cells by estrogen and phytoestrogens. *J Biol Chem* 280:13720-13727.

[172] Karieb S, Fox SW (2011) Phtoestrogens directly inhibit TNF-α-induced bone resorption in RAW264.7 cells by suppressing c-fos-induced NFATc1 expression. *J Cell Biochem* 112:476-487.

[173] Gao YH, Yamaguchi M (1999) Suppressive effect of genistein on rat bone osteoclasts: Apoptosis is induced through Ca^{2+} signaling. *Biol Pharm Bull* 22: 805-809.

[174] Gao YH, Yamaguchi M (2000) Suppressive effect of genistein on rat bone osteoclasts: Involvement of protein kinase inhibition and protein tyrosine phosphatase activation. *Int J Mol Med* 5: 261-267.

[175] Murrills RJ, Shane E, Lindsay R, Dempster DW (1989) Bone resorption by isolated human osteoclasts in vitro: effects of calcitonin. *J Bone Miner Res* 4: 259-268.

[176] Su Y, Charkrabort M, Nathanson MH, Baron R (1992) Differential effects of the 3', 5'-cyclic adenosine moncphosphate and proein kinase C pathways on the response of isolated rat osteoclasts to calcitonin. *Endocrinology* 131: 1497-1502.

[177] Jones DOP, McConkey DJ, Nicotera P, Orrenius S (1989) Calcium-activated DNA fragmentation in rat liver nuclei. *J Biol Chem* 264: 6398-6403.

[178] McCabe MJ, Orrenius S (1993) Genistein induces apoptosis in immature human thymocytes by inhibiting topoisomerase-II. *Biochem Biophys Res Commun* 194: 944-950.

[179] Missbach M, Jeschke M, Feyen J, Muller K, Glatt M, Green J, Susa M (1999) A novel inhibitor of the tyrosine kinase Src suppresses phosphoryalation of its major cellular substrates and reduces bone resorption in vitro and in rodent models *in vivo*. *Bone* 24: 437-449.

[180] Hunter T (1995) Protein kinases and phosphatases: the Yin and Yang of protein phosphorylation and signaling. *Cell* 80: 225-236.

[181] Aoki K, Didomenico E, Sims NA, Mukhopadhyay K, Neff L, Houghton A, Amling M, Levy JB, Horne WC, Baron R (1999) The tyrosine phosphatase SHP-1 is a negative regulator of osteoclastogenesis and osteoclast resorbing activity: increased resorption and osteopenia in $me^{v}.me^{v}$ mutant mice. *Bone* 25: 261-267.

[182] Uchiyama S, Yamaguchi M (2007) Genistein and zinc synergistically stimulate apoptotic cell death and suppress RANKL siganling-related gene expression in osteoclastic cells. *J Cell Biochem* 101: 529-542.

[183] Ono R, Yamaguchi M (1999) Increase in bone components of rats orally administered isoflavone-containing soybean extract *(Nijiru)*. *J Health Sci* 45: 66-69.

[184] Ono R, Yamaguchi M (1999) Anabolic effect of soybean saponin on bone components in the femoral tissues of rats. *J Health Sci* 45: 251-255.

[185] Ono R, Ma ZJ, Yamaguchi M (2000) Prolonged intake of fermented soybean diets with supplementation of isoflavone and saponin prevents bone loss in ovariectomized rats. *J Health Sci* 46: 70 -74.

[186] Gallo D, Zannoni GF, Apollon P, Martinelli E, Ferlin C, Passetti G, Riva A, Morazzoni P, Bombardelli E, Scambia G (2005) Characterization of the pharmacologic profile rat model of menopause: effects on bone, uterus, and lipid profile. *Menopause* 12:589-600.

[187] Yamaguchi M, Ono R, Ma ZJ (2001) Prolonged intake of isoflavone- and saponin-containing soybean extract *(nijiru)* supplement enhances circulating γ-carboxylated osteocalcin concentration in healthy individuals. *J Health Sci* 47: 579-58239.

[188] Yamaguchi M, Igarashi A, Sakai M, Degawa H, Ozawa Y (2005) Prolonged intake of dietary fermented isoflavone-rich soybean reinforced with zinc affects circulating bone biochemical markers in aged individuals. *J Health Sci* 51: 191-196.

[189] Ma ZJ, Shimanuki S, Igarashi A, Kawasaki Y, Yamaguchi M (2000) Preventive effect of dietary fermented soybean on bone loss in ovariectomized rats: Enhancement with isoflavone and zinc supplementation. *J Health Sci* 46: 263-268.

[190] Gao YH, Yamaguchi M (1998) Zinc enhancement of genistein's anabolic effect on bone components in elderly female rats. *Gen Pharmacol* 31:199-202.

[191] Yamaguchi M, Gao YH, Ma ZJ (2000) Synergistic effect of genistein and zinc on bone components in the femoral-metaphyseal tissues of female rats. *J Bone Miner Metab* 18: 77-83.

[192] Ma ZJ, Igarashi A, Inagaki M, Mitsugi F, Yamaguchi M (2000) Supplemental intake of isoflavones and zinc-containing mineral mixture enhances bone components in the femoral tissues of rats with increasing age. *J Health Sci* 46: 363-369.

[193] Uchiyama S, Yamaguchi M (2007) Genistein and zinc synergistically enhance gene expression and mineralization in osteoblastic MC3T3-E1 cells. *Int J Mol Med* 19: 213-220.

[194] Uchiyama S, Yamaguchi M (2007) Genistein and zinc synergistically stimulate apoptotic cell death and suppress RANKL signlaing-related gene expression in osteoclastic cells. *J Cell Biochem* 101: 529-542.

[195] Kim K, Kim JH, Lee J, Jim HM, Lee SH, Fisher DE, Kook H, Kim KK, Choi Y, Kim N (2005) Nuclear factor of activated T cells c1 induces osteoclast-associated receptor gene expression during tumor necrosis factor-related activation-induced cytokine-mediated osteoclastogenesis. *J Biol Chem* 280: 35209-35216.

[196] Ma ZJ, Shimanuki S, Igarashi A, Kawasaki Y, Yamaguchi M (2000) Preventive effect of dietary fermented soybean on bone loss in ovariectomized rats: Enhancement with isoflavone and zinc supplementation. *J Health* Sci 46: 263-268.

[197] Yamaguchi M, Igarashi A, Sakai M, Degawa H, Ozawa Y (2005) Prolonged intake of dietary fermented isoflavone-rich soybean reinforced with zinc affects circulating bone biochemical markers in aged individuals. *J Health Sci* 51: 191-196.

[198] Iwamoto J, Sato Y, Takeda T, Matumoto H (2009) High-dose vitamin K supplementation reduces fracture incidence in postmenopausal women: a review of the literature. *Nutr Res* 29, 221-228.

[199] Koshihara Y, Hoshi K, Shiraki M (1992) Enhancement of mineralization of human osteoblasts by vitamin K_2 (menaquinone-4). *J Clin Exp Med* 161: 439-440.

[200] Hauschka PV, Lian JB, Gallop PM (1975) Direct identification of the calcium-binding amino acid, γ-carboxyglutamate, in mineralized tissue. *Proc Natl Acad Sci* USA 72: 3925-3929.

[201] Price PA (1985) Vitamin K-dependent formation of bone gla protein (osteocalcin) and its function. *Vitam Horm* 42: 65-108.

[202] Hauschka PV, Carr SA (1982) Calcium-dependent α-helical structure in osteocalcin. *Biochemistry* 21: 2538-2547.

[203] Akiyama Y, Hara K, Ohkawa I, Tajima, T (1993) Effects of menaterenone on bone loss induced by ovariectomy in rats. *Jpn J Pharmacol* 62: 145-153.

[204] Hosoi T (1996) Recent progress in treatement of osteoporosis. *Nippon Ronnen Igaku Zasshi* 33: 240-244.

[205] Ehara Y, Takahashi H, Hanahisa Y, Yamaguchi M (1996) Effect of vitamin K_2 (menaquinone-7) on bone metabolism in the femoral-metaphyseal tissues of normal and skeletal-unloaded rats: enhancement with zinc. *Res Exp Med* 196: 171-178.

[206] Yamaguchi M, Uchiyama S, Tsukamoto Y (2002) Stimulatory effect of menaquinone-7 on bone formation in elderly female rat femoral tissues *in vitro*: Prevention of bone deterioration with aging. *Int J Mol Med* 10: 720-733.

[207] Knapen MHJ, Hamulyak K, Vermeer C (1989) The effect of vitamin K supplementation on circulating osteocalcin (bone gla protein) and urinary calcium excretion. *Ann Intern Med* 111: 1001-1005.

[208] Hart JP, Sheaver MJ, Klenerman L, Catterall A, Reeve J, Sambrook PN, Dodds, RA, Bitensky L, Chayen J (1985) Electrochemical detection of depressed circulating levels of vitamin K_1 in osteoporosis. *J Clin Endocrinol Metab* 60:1268-1269.

[209] Yamaguchi M (2002) Isoflavone and bone metabolism: Its cellular mechanism and preventive role in bone loss. *J Health Sci* 48: 209-222.

[210] Yamaguchi M, Gao-Balch Y (2013) Role of dietary soybean genistein in osteoporosis prevention. *Int J Food Sci Nutr Dietetics* 2:102.

[211] Yamaguchi M (2006) Regulatory mechanism of food factors in bone metabolism and prevention of osteoporosis. *Yakugaku Zasshi* 126: 1117-1137.

[212] Yamaguchi M (2012) Nutritional factors and bone homeostasis: synergistic effect of zinc and genistein in osteogenesis. *Mol Cell Biochem* 366:201-221.

[213] Shearer M J (2009) Vitamin K in parenteral nutrition. *Gastroenterology* 137:S105-S118.

[214] Shearer MJ (2000). Role of vitamin K and Gla proteins in the pathophysiology of oetoporosis and vascular calcification. *Cur Opin Clin Nutr Metab Care* 3: 433-438.

[215] Schurgers LJ, Teunissen KJF, Hamulyak K, Knapen MHJ, Vik H, Vermeer G (2007) Vitamin K-containing dietary supplements: comparison of synthetic vitamin K_1 and natto-derived menaquinone-7. *Blood* 109: 3279-3283.

[216] Schurgers LJ, Vermeer C (2000) Determination of phyloquinone and menaquinones in food: effect of food matrix on circulating vitamin K concentrations. *Haemostasis* 30: 298-307.

[217] Schurgers LJ, Vermeer C (2002) Differential lipoprotein transport pathways of K-vitamins in healthy subjects. *Biochim Biophys Acta* 1570: 27-32.

[218] Delmas PD (1993) Biochemical markers of bone turnover. 1. Theoretical considerations and clinical use in osteoporosis. *Am J Med* 95 (suppl 5A): 11-16.

[219] Miki T, Nakatsuka K, Naka H, Kitatani K, Saito S, Masaki H, Tomiyoshi Y, Morii H, Nishizawa Y (2003) Vitamin K_2 (menaquinone 4) reduces serum undercarboxylated osteocalcin level as early as 2 weeks in elderly women with established osteoporosis. *J Bone Miner Metab* 21: 161-165.

[220] Van Summeren MJH, Braam LAJ, Lilien MR, Schurgers LJ, Kuis W, Vermeer C (2009) The effect of menaquinone-7 (vitamin K_2) supplementation on osteocalcin carboxylation in healthy prepubertal children. *Brit J Nutr* 102: 1171-1178.

[221] Koshihara Y, Hosoi K (1997) Vitamin K_2 enhances osteocalcin accumulation in the extracellular matrix of human osteoblasts in vitro. *J Bone Miner Res* 12: 431-438.

[222] Hodges SJ, Akesson K, Vergnaud P, Obrant K, Delmas PD (1993) Circulating levels of vitamin K_1 and K_2 decreased in elderly woman with hip fracture. *J Bone Miner Res* 8: 1241-1245.

[223] Binkley NC, Krueger DC, Engelke JA, Foley AL, Suttie JW (2000) VitaminK supplementation reduces serum concentrations of under-gamma-carboxylated osteocalcin in healthy young and elderly adults. *Am J Clin Nutr* 72: 1523-1528.

[224] Knapen MHJ, Jie KSG, Hamulyak K, Vermeer C (1993) VitaminK-induced changes in markers for osteoblast activity and urinary calcium loss. *Calcif Tissue Int* 53: 81-85.

[225] Schaafsma A, Muskiet FA, Storm H, Hofstede GJ, Pakan I, Van der Veer E (2000). Vitamin D_3 and vitamin K_1 supplementation of Dutch postmenopausal women with normal and low bone mineral densities: effects on serum 25-hydroxyvitamin D and carboxylated osteocalcin. *Eur J Clin Nutr* 54: 626-631.

[226] Yamaguchi M, Sugimoto E, Hachiya S (2001) Stimulatory effect of menaquinone-7 (vitamin K_2) on osteoblastic bone formation *in vitro*. *Mol Cell Biochem* 223: 131-137.

[227] Yamaguchi M, Ma ZJ (2001) Inhibitory effect of menaquinone-7 (vitamin K_2) on osteoclast-like cell formation and osteoclastic bone resorption in rat bone tissues *in vitro*. *Mol Cell Biochem* 228: 39-47.

[228] Yamaguchi M, Weitzmann MN (2011) Vitamin K_2 stimulates osteoblastogenesis and suppresses osteoclastogenesis by suppressing NF-κB activation. *Int J Mol Med* 27: 3-14.

[229] Tabb MM, Sun A, Zhou C, Grun F, Errandi J, Romero K, Pham H, Inoue S, Mallick S, Lin, Forman BM, Blumberg B (2003) Vitamin K_2 regulation of bone homeostasis is mediated by the steroid and xenobiotic receptor SXR. *J Biol Chem* 278:43919-43927.

[230] Yamaguchi M, Taguchi H, Gao YH, Igarashi A, Tsukamoto Y (1999) Effect of vitamin K_2 (menaquinone-7) in fermented soybean (*natto*) on bone loss in ovariectomized rats. *J Bone Miner Metab* 17: 23-29.

[231] Yamaguchi M, Kakuda H, Gao YH, Tsukamoto Y (2000) Prolonged intake of fermented soybean (*natto*) diets containing vitamin K_2 (menaquinone-7) prevents bone loss in ovariectomized rats. *J Bone Miner Metab* 18: 71-76.

[232] Ma ZJ, Igarashi A, Yamakawa K, Yamaguchi M (2001) Enhancing effect of zinc and vitamin K_2 (menaquinone-7) on bone components in the femoral tissues of female elderly rats. *J Health Sci* 47: 40-45.

[233] Tsukamoto Y, Ichise H, Yamaguchi M (2000) Prolonged intake of dietary fermented soybeans (*natto*) with the reinforced vitamin K_2 (menaquinone-7) enhances circulating γ-carboxylated osteocalcin concentration in normal individuals. *J Health Sci* 46:317-321.

[234] Tsukamoto Y, Ichise H, Kakuda K, Yamaguchi M (2000) Intake of fermented soybean (*natto*) increases circulating vitamin K_2 (menaquinone-7) and γ-carboxylated osteocalcin concentration in normal individuals. *J Bone Miner Metab* 18:216-222.

[235] Knapen MHJ, Drummen NE, Smit E, Vermeer C, Theuwissen E (2013) Three-year low-dose menaquinone-7 supplementation helps decrease bone loss healthy postmenopausal women. *Osteoporosis Int,* doi 10.1007/s00198-013-2325-6.

[236] Williams JA, Kondo N, Okabe T, Takeshita N, Pilchak DM, Koyama E, Ochiai T, Jensen D, Chu M-L, Kane MA, Napoli JL, Enomoto-Iwamoto M, Ghyselinck N, Chambon P, Pacifici M, Iwamoto M (2009) Retinoic acid receptors are required for skeletal growth, matrix homeostasis and growth plate function in postnatal mouse. *Dev Biol* 328, 315-327.

[237] Park CK, Ishimi Y, Ohmura M, Yamaguchi M, Ikegami S (1997) Vitamin A and carotenoids stimulate differentiation of mouse osteoblastic cells. *J Nutr Sci Vitaminol* (Tokyo). 43, 281-296.

[238] Conaway H H, Persson E, Halén M, Granholm S, Svensson O, Pettersson U, Lie A, Lerner UH (2009) Retinoids inhibit differentiation of hematopoetic osteoclast progenitors. *FASEB J* 23, 3526-3538.

[239] Promislow JHE, Goodman-Gruen D, Slymen DJ, Barret-Connor E (2002) Retinol intake and bone mineral density in the elderly: the rancho brenardo study. *J Bone Miner Res* 17:1349-1358.

[240] Mata-Granados JM, Cuenca-Acevedo R, Luque de Castro MD, Sosa M, Quesada-Gómez JM (2010) Vitamin D deficiency and high serum levels of vitamin A increase the risk of osteoporosis evaluated by Quantitative Ultrasound Measurements (QUS) in postmenopausal Spanish women. *Clin Biochem* 43: 1064-1068.

[241] Ribaya-Mercado JD, Blumberg JB (2007) Vitamin A: is it a risk factor for osteoporosis and bone fracture? *Nutr Rev* 65: 425-38.

[242] Maggio D, Polidori MC, Barabani M, Tufi A, Ruggiero C, Cecchetti R, Aisa MC, Stahl W, Cherubini A (2006) Low levels of carotenoids and retinol in involutional osteoporosis. *Bone* 38: 244-248.

[243] Yamaguchi M, Uchiyama S (2003) Effect of carotenoid on calcium content and alkaline phosphatase activity in rat femoral tissues in vitro: The unique anabolic effect of β-cryptoxanthin. *Biol Pharm Bull* 26: 1188-1191.

[244] Yamaguchi M, Uchiyama S (2004) β-Cryptoxanthin stimulates bone formation and inhibits bone resorption in tissue culture *in vitro*. *Mol Cell Biochem* 258: 137-144.

[245] Rao LG, Krishnadev N, Banasikowska K, Rao AV (2003) Lycopene effects on osteoclasts: lycopene inhibits basal and parathyroid hormone-stimulated osteoclast formation and mineral resorption mediated by reactive oxygen species in rat bone marrow cultures. *J Med Food* 6: 69-78.

[246] Rao LG, Mackinnon ES, Josse RG, Murray T M, Strauss A, Rao A V (2007) Lycopene consumption decreases oxidative stress and bone resorption markers in postmenopausal women. *Osteoporos Int* 18: 109-115.

[247] Mackinnon ES, Rao AV, Josse RG, Rao L G (2011) Supplementation with the antioxidant lycopene significantly decreases oxidative stress parameters and the bone resorption marker N-telopeptide of type I collagen in postmenopausal women. *Osteoporos Int* 22:1091-1101.

[248] Caire-Juvera G, Ritenbaugh C, Wactawski-Wende J, Snetselaar LG, Chen Z (2009) Vitamin A and retinol intakes and the risk of fractures among participants of the Women's Health Initiative Observational Study. *Am J Clin Nutr* 89: 323-30.

[249] McEligot AJ, Rock CL, Shanks TG, Flatt SW, Newman V, Farber S, Pierce JP (1999) Comparison of serum carotenoid responses between women consuming vegetable juice and women consuming raw or cooked vegetable. *Cancer Epideminol Biomarkers Prev* 8: 227-231.

[250] Uchiyama S, Yamaguchi M (2005) β-Cryptoxanthin stimulates cell proliferation and transcriptional activity in osteoblastic MC3T3-E1cells. *Int J Mol Med* 15: 675-681.

[251] Uchiyama S, Yamaguchi M (2005) β-Cryptoxanthin stimulates cell differentiation and mineralization in osteoblastic MC3T3-E1 cells. *J Cell Biochem* 95: 1224-1234.

[252] Centrella M, McCarthy TL, Canalis E (1990) Receptors for insulin-like growth factor-I and -II in osteoblast-enriched cultures from fetal rat bone. *Endocrinology* 126:39-44.

[253] Palcy S, Bolivar I, Goltzman D (2000) Role of activator protein 1 transcriptional activity in the regulation of gene expression by transforming growth factor β1 and bone morphogenic protein 2 in ROS 17/2.8 osteoblast-like cells. *J Bone Miner Res* 15: 2352-2361.

[254] Komori T, Yagi H, Nomura S, Yamaguchi A, Sasaki K, Deguchi K, Shimizu Y, Bronson RT, Gao YH, Inada M, Sato M, Okamoto R, Kitamura Y, Yoshiki S, Kishimoto T (1997) Targeted disruption of Cbfa1 results in a comple lack of bone formation owing to maturational arrest of osteoblasts. *Cell* 89: 755-764.

[255] Yohay DA, Zhang J, Thrailkill KM, Arthur JM, Quarles LD (1994) Role of serum in the developmental expression of alkaline phosphatase in MC3T3-E1 osteoblasts. *J Cell Physiol* 158: 467-475.

[256] Uchiyama S, Yamaguchi M (2004) Inhibitory effect of β -cryptoxanthin on osteoclast-like cell formation in mouse marrow cultures. *Biochem Pharmacol* 67: 1297-1305.

[257] Anderson DM, Maraskovsky E, Billingsley WL, Dougall WC, Tometsko ME, Roux ER, Teepe MC, DuBose RF, Cosman D, Gailibert L (1997) A homologue of the TNF receptor and its ligand enhance T-cell growth and dendritic-cell function. *Nature* 390: 175-195.

[258] Lee ZH, Kwack K, Kim K K, Lee SH, Kim H-H (2000) Activation of c-Jun N-terminal kinase and activator protein 1 by receptor activator of NF-κB. *Mol Pharmacol* 58: 1536-1545.

[259] Uchiyama S, Yamaguchi M (2006) β-Cryptoxanthin stimulates apoptotic cell death and suppresses cell function in osteoclastic cells: Change in their related gene expression. *J Cell Biochem* 98: 1185-1195.

[260] Uchiyama S, Ishiyama K, Hashimoto K, Yamaguchi M (2005) Synergistic effect of β-cryptoxanthin and zinc sulfate on the bone component in rat femoral tissues *in vitro*: The unique anabolic effect with zinc. *Biol Pharm Bull* 28: 2142-2145.

[261] Uchiyama S, Yamaguchi M (2008) Anabolic effect of β-cryptoxanthin in osteoblastic MC3T3-E1 cells is enhanced with 17 β-estradiol, genistein, or zinc sulfate in vitro: the unique effect with zinc on Runx2 and α1(I) collagen mRNA espression. *Mol Cell Biochem* 307: 209-219.

[262] Yamaguchi M, Uchiyama S (2008) Combination of β -cryptoxanthin and zinc has potent effects on apoptotic cell death and suppression of bone resorption-related gene expression in osteoclastic cells. *Int J Mol Med* 22: 221-228.

[263] Yamaguchi M, Uchiyama S, Ishiyama K, Hashimoto K (2006) Oral administration in combination with zinc enhances β-cryptoxanthin-induced anabolic effects on bone components in the femoral tissues of rats *in vivo*. *Biol Pharm Bull* 29: 371-374.

[264] Uchiyama S, Sumida T, Yamaguchi M (2004) Oral administration of β-cryptoxanthin induces anabolic effects on bone components in the femoral tissues of rats *in vivo*. *Biol Pharm Bull* 27: 232-235.

[265] Uchiyama S, Sumida T, Yamaguchi M (2004) Anabolic effect of β-cryptoxanthin on bone components in the femoral tissues of aged rats *in vivo* and *in vitro*. *J Health Sci* 50: 491- 496.

[266] Uchiyama S, Yamaguchi M (2005) Oral administration of β-cryptoxanthin prevents bone loss in streptozotocin-diabetic rats *in vivo*. *Biol Pharm Bull* 28: 1766-1769.

[267] Uchiyama S, Yamaguchi M (2006) Oral administration of β-cryptoxanthin prevents bone loss in ovariectomized rats. *Int J Mol Med* 17: 15-20.

[268] Price PA (1985) Vitamin K-dependent formation of bone gla protein (osteocalcin) and its function. *Vitam Horm* 42: 65-108.

[269] Levy JR, Murray E, Manolagass S, Olefsky JM (1986) Demonstration of insulin receptors and modulation of alkaline phosphatase activity by insulin in rat osteoblastic cells. *Endocrinology* 119: 1786-1792.

[270] Hallen JM, Alatalo SL, Suminen H, Cheng S, Janekila A., &Vaananen, H K (2000) Tartrate-resistant acid phosphatase 5b: A novel serum marker of bone resorption. *J Bone Miner Res* 15: 1337-1345.

[271] Clements JD, Herrick MV, Singer FR, Eyre DR (1997) Evidence that serum NTx (collagen-type I N-telopeptides) can act as an immunochemical marker of bone resorption. *Clin Chem* 43: 2058-2063.

[272] Yamaguchi M, Igarashi A, Uchiyama S, Morita S, Sugawara K, Sumida K (2004) Prolonged intake of jucice (*Citrus unshiu*) reinforced with β-cryptoxanthin has an effect on circulating bone biochemical markers in normal individuals. *J Health Sci* 50: 619-624.

[273] Yamaguchi M, Igarashi A, Morita S, Sumida T, Sugawara K (2005) Relationship between serum β-cryptoxanthin and circulating bone metabolic markers in healthy individuals with the intake of juice (*Citrus unshiu*) containing β-cryptoxanthin. *J Health Sci* 51: 738-743.

[274] Yamaguchi M, Igarashi A, Uchiyama S, Sugawara K, Sumida T, Morita S, Ogawa H, Nishitani M, Kajimoto Y (2006) Effect of β-cryptoxanthin on circulating bone metabolic markers: Intake of juice (*Citrus unshiu*) supplemented with β-cryptoxanthin has an effect in menopausal women. *J Health Sci* 52: 758-768.

[275] Wang Y, Hodge AM, Wluka AE, English DR, Giles GG, O'Sullivan R, Forbes A, Cicuttini FM (2007) Effect of antioxidants on knee cartilage and bone in healthy, middle-aged subjects: a cross-sectional study. *Arthritis Res Ther* 9: R66.

[276] Sugiura M, Nakamura M, Ogawa K, Ikoma Y, Ando F, Yano M (2008) Bone mineral density in post-menopausal female subjects is associated with serum antioxidant carotenoids. *Osteoporos Int* 19: 211-219-720.

[277] Sugiura M, Nakamura M, Ogawa K, Ikoma Y, Yano M (2012) High serum carotenoids associated with lower risk for bone loss and osteoporosis in post-menopausal Japanese female subjects: prospective cohort study. *PLoS One* 7: e52643. doi: 10.1371/journal.pone.0052643.

[278] Granado-Lorencio F, Olmedilla-Alonso B, Herrero-Barbudo C, Blanco-Navarro I, Perez-Sacristan B (2008) Seasonal variation of serum alpha- and beta-cryptoxanthin and 25-OH-vitamin D_3 in women with osteoporosis. *Osteoporos Int* 19: 717-720.

[279] Sahni S, Hannan MT, Blumberg J, Cupples LA, Kiel DP, Tucker KL (2009) Protective effect of total carotenoid and lycopene intake on the risk of hip fracture: A 17-year follow-up from the Framingham osteoporosis study. *J Bone Miner Res* 24: 1086-1094.

[280] Yang Z, Zhang Z, Penniston KL, Binkley N, Tanumihardjo SA (2008) Serum carotenoid concentrations in postmenopausal women from the United States with and without osteoporosis. *Int J Vitm Nutr Res* 78; 105-110.

[281] Sugiura M, Nakamura M, Ogawa K, Ikoma Y, Ando F, Shimokata H, Yano M (2010) Dietary patterns of antioxidant vitamin and carotenoid intake associated with bone mineral density: findings from post-menopausal Japanese female subjects. Osteoporos Int 36:2293-2298.

[282] Lai YL, Yamaguchi M (2006) Phytocomponent *p*-hydroxycinnamic acid stimulates bone formation and inhibits bone resorption in rat femoral tissues *in vitro*. *Mol Cell Biochem* 292: 45-52.

[283] Yamaguchi M, Lai YL, Uchiyama S, Nakagawa T (2008) Phytocomponent *p*-hydroxycinnamic acid stimulates mineralization in osteoblastic MC3T3-E1 cells. *Int J Mol Med* 22: 287-291.

[284] Nanes MS (2003) Tumor necrosis factor-alpha: molecular and cellular mechanisms in skeletal pathology. *Gene* 321: 1-15.

[285] Teti A Colucci S, Grano M, Argentino L, Zallone AZ (1992) Protein kinase C afftects microfilaments, bone resorption, and [Ca^{2+}] sensing in cultured osteoclasts. *Am J Physiol 263:C130-C139.*

[286] Franzoso G, Carlson L, Xing L, Poljak L, shores EW, Brown KD, Leonardi A, Tran T, Boyce BF, Siebenlist U (1997) Requirement for NF-kappaB in osteoclast and B-cell development. *Genes Dev* 11: 3482-3496.

[287] Boyce BF, Xing L, Franzoso G and Siebenlist U (1999) Required and nonessential functions of nuclear factor-kappa B in bone cells. *Bone* 25: 137-139.

[288] Lai YL, Yamaguchi M (2007) Phytocomponent *p*-hydroxycinnamic acid inhibits osteoclast-like cell formation in mouse bone marrow cultures. *Int J Mol Med* 19: 123-128.

[289] Iotsova V, Caamano J, Loy J, Yang Y, Lewin A, Bravo R (1997) Osteopetrosis in mice lacking NF-kappaB1 and NF-kappaB2. *Nat Med* 3: 1285-1289.

[290] Li Y, Li A, Strait K, Zhang H, Nanes MS and Weitzmann MN (2007) Endogenous TNFalpha Lowers Maximum Peak Bone Mass and Inhibits Osteoblastic Smad Activation, through NF-kappaB. *J Bone Miner Res* 22: 646-655.

[291] Eliseev RA, Schwarz EM, Zuscik MJ, O'Keefe RJ, Drissi H, Rosier RN (2006) Smad7 mediates inhibition of Saos2 osteosarcoma cell differentiation by NFkappaB. *Exp Cell Res* 312: 40-50.

[292] Yamaguchi M, Weitzmann MN (2009) The bone anabolic carotenoids *p*-hydroxycinnamic acid and β-cryptoxanthin antagonize NF-κB activation in MC3T3 preosteoblasts. *Mol Med Reports* 2:641-644.

[293] Yamaguchi M, Weitzmann MN (2012) The bone anabolic carotenoid *p*-hydroxycinnamic acid promotes osteoblast mineralization and suppresses osteoclast differentiation by antagonizing NF-κB activation. *Int J Mol Med* 30:708-712.

[294] Vaira S, Alhawagri M, Anwisye I, Kitaura H, Faccio R, Novack DV (2008) RelA/p65 promotes osteoclast differentiation by blocking a RANKL-induced apoptotic JNK pathway in mice. *J Clin Invest* 118: 2088-2097.

[295] Lai YL, Yamaguchi M (2006) Oral administration of phytocomponent *p*-hydroxycinnamic acid has anabolic effects on bone calcification in femoral tissues of rats *in vivo*. *J Health Sci 52*: 308-312.

[296] Minkin C (1982) Bone acid phosphatase: tartrate-resistant acid phosphatase as a marker of osteoclast function. *Calcif Tissue Int* 34:285-290.

[297] Chen J-R, Lazarenko OP, Wu X, Kang J, Blackburn ML, Shankar K, Badger TM, Ronis MJJ (2010) Dietary-induced serum phenolic acids promote bone growth via p38 MAPK/β-catenin canonical Wnt signaling. *J Bone Miner Res* 25:2399-2411.

[298] Yamaguchi M, Lai YL, Uchiyama S, Nakagawa T (2008) Oral administration of phytocomponent *p*-hydroxycinnamic acid prevents bone loss in ovariectomized rats. *Mol Cell Biochem* 311: 31-36.

[299] Shires R, Teitelbaum SL, Bergfeld MA, Fallom MD, Statopolsky E, Avioli LV (1981) The effect of streptozotocin-induced chronic diabetes mellitus on bone and mineral homeostasis in the rat. *J Lab Clin Med* 97:231-240.

[300] Leslie WD, Rubin MR, Schwartz AV, Kanis JA (2012) Type 2 diabetes and bone. *J Bone Miner Res* 27:2231-2237.

[301] Lai YL, Yamaguchi M (2007) Oral administration of phytocomponent *p*-hydroxycinnamic acid has a preventive effect on bone loss in streptozotocin-induced diabetic rats. *Int J Mol Med* 19: 803-807.

[302] Nyomba BL, verhaeghe J, thomasser M, Lissens W, Bouillon R (1980) Bone mineral homeostasis in spontaneously diabetic BB rats. I. Abnormal vitamin D metabolism and impaired active intestinal calcium absorption. *Endocrinology* 124:565-572.

[303] Yamaguchi M, Hamamoto R, Uchiyama S, Ishiyama K (2007) Effects of flavonoid on calcium content in femoral tissue culture and parathyroid hormone-stimulated osteoclastogenesis in bone marrow culture in vitro. *Mol Cell Biochem* 303: 83-88.

[304] Wattel A, Kamel S, Prouillet C, Petti JP, Lorget F, Offord E, Brazier M (2004) Flavonoid qyercetin decreases osteoclastic differentiation induced by RANKL via a mechanism involving NF kappa B and AP-1. *J Cell Biochem* 15:285-295.

[305] Cheng WC, Huang RY, Chiang CY, Chen JK, Liu CH, Chu CL, Fu E (2010) Ameliorative effect of quercetin on the destruction caused by experimental periodontitis in rats. *J Periodontal Res* 45: 788-795.

[306] Hamalainen M, Nieminen R, Vuorela P, Heinonen M, Moilanen E (2007) Anti-inflammatory effects of flavonoids: genistein, kaempferol, quercetin, and daidzein inhibit STAT-1 and NF-kappaB activations, whereas flavone, isorhamnetin, naringenin, and pelargonidin inhibit only NF-kappaB activation along with their inhibitory effect on iNOS expression and NO production in activated macrophages. *Mediators Inflamm* 2007: 45673. doi: 10.1155/2007/45673.

[307] Nam NH (2006) Naturally occurring NF-kappaB inhibitors. *Mini Rev Med* Chem 6: 945-951.

[308] Leibbrandt A, Penninger JM (2009) RANKL/RANK as key factors for osteoclast development and bone loss in arthropaties. *Adv Exp Med Biol* 649:100-113.

[309] Xing L, Bushnell TP, Carlson L, Tai Z, Tondravi M, Siebenlist U, Young F, Boyce BF (2002) NF-kappaB p50 and p52 expression is not required for RANK-expressing osteoclast progenitor formation but is essential for RANK- and cytokine-mediated osteoclastogenesis. *J Bone Miner Res* 17: 1200-1210.

[310] Vaira S, Johnson T, Hirbe AC, Alhawaqri M, Anwisye I, Sammut B, O'Neal J, Zou W, Weilbaecher KN, Faccio R, Novack DV (2008) RelB is the NF-kappaB subunit downstream of NIK responsible for osteoclast differentiation. *Proc Natl Acad Sci U S A* 105: 3897-3902.

[311] Boyce BF, Yao Z, Xing L (2010) Functions of nuclear factor kappaB in bone. *Ann N Y Acad Sci* 1192: 367-375.

[312] Woo JT, Nakagawa H, Notoya M, Yonezawa T, Udagawa N, Lee IS, Ohnishi M, Hagiwara H, Nagai K (2004) Quercetin suppresses bone resorption by inhibiting the differentiation and activation of osteoclasts. *Biol Pharm Bull* 27: 504-509.

[313] Wattel A, Kamel S, Mentaverri R, Lorget F, Prouillet C, Petti JP, Fardelonne P, Brazier M (2003) Potent inhibitory effect of naturally occurring flavonoids quercetin and kaempferol on in vitro osteoclastic bone resorption. *Biochem Pharmacol* 65: 35-42.

[314] Wattel A, Kamel S, Prouillet C, Petit JP, Lorget F, Offord E, Brazier M (2004) Flavonoid quercetin decreases osteoclastic differentiation induced by RANKL via a mechanism involving NF kappa B and AP-1. *J Cell Biochem* 92: 285-295.

[315] Siddiqui JA, Sharan K, Swarnkar G, Rawat P, Kumar M, Manickavasagam L, Maurya R, Pierroz D, Chattopadhyay N (2011) Quercetin-6-C-beta-D-glucopyranoside isolated from Ulmus wallichiana planchon is more potent than quercetin in inhibiting osteoclastogenesis and mitigating ovariectomy-induced bone loss in rats. *Menopause* 18: 198-207.

[316] Chang J, Wang Z, Tang E, Fan Z, McCauley L, Franceschi R, Guan K, Krebsbach PH, Wang CY (2009) Inhibition of osteoblastic bone formation by nuclear factor-kappaB. *Nat Med* 15: 682-689.

[317] Alles N, Soysa NS, Hayashi J, Khan M, Shimoda A, Shimokawa H, Ritzeler O, Akiyoshi K, Aoki K, Ohya K (2010) Suppression of NF-kappaB increases bone formation and ameliorates osteopenia in ovariectomized mice. *Endocrinology* 151: 4626-4634.

[318] Wahl EC, Aronson J, Liu L,Fowlkes JL, Thrailkill KM, Bunn RC, Skinner RA, Miller MJ, Cockrell GE, Clark LM, Ou Y, Isales CM, Badger TM, Ronis MJ, Sims J, Lumpkin CK Jr (2010) Restoration of Regenerative Osteoblastogenesis in Aged Mice: Modulation of TNF. *J Bone Miner Res* 25: 114-123.

[319] Notoya M, Tsukamoto Y, Nishimura H, Woo JT, Nagai K, Lee IS, Hagiwara H (2004) Quercetin, a flavonoid, inhibits the proliferation, differentiation, and mineralization of osteoblasts in vitro. *Eur J Pharmacol* 485: 89-96.

[320] Son YO, Kook SH, Choi KC, Jang YS, Jeon YM, Kim JG, Lee KY, Kim J, Chung MS, Chung GH, Lee JC (2006) Quercetin, a bioflavonoid, accelerates TNF-alpha-induced growth inhibition and apoptosis in MC3T3-E1 osteoblastic cells. *Eur J Pharmacol* 529: 24-32.

[321] Nam TW, Yoo CI, Kim HT, Kwon CH, Park JY, Kim YK (2008) The flavonoid quercetin induces apoptosis and inhibits migration through a MAPK-dependent mechanism in osteoblasts. *J Bone Miner Metab* 26: 551-560.

[322] Prouillet C, Maziere JC, Maziere C, Wattel A, Brazier M, Kamel S (2004) Stimulatory effect of naturally occurring flavonols quercetin and kaempferol on alkaline phosphatase activity in MG-63 human osteoblasts through ERK and estrogen receptor pathway. *Biochem Pharmacol* 67: 1307-1313.

[323] Yamaguchi M, Weitzmann MN (2011) Quercetin, a potent suppressor NF-κB and Smad activation in osteoblasts. *Int J Mol Med* 28:521-525.

[324] Janssens K, Ten Dijke P, Janssens S, Van Hul W (2005) Transforming Growth Factor-{beta}1 to the Bone. *Endocr Rev* 26: 743-774.

[325] Canalis E, Economides AN, Gazzerro E (2003) Bone morphogenetic proteins, their antagonists, and the skeleton. *Endocr Rev* 24: 218-235.

[326] Phan TT, Lim IJ, Chan SY, Tan EK, Lee ST, Longaker MT (2004) Suppression of transforming growth factor beta/smad signaling in keloid-derived fibroblasts by quercetin: implications for the treatment of excessive scars. *J Trauma* 57: 1032-1037.

[327] Tsuji M, Yamamoto H, Sato T, Mizuha Y, Kawai Y, Taketani Y, Kato S, Terao J, Inakuma T, Takeda E (2009) Dietary qyercetin inhibits bone loss without effect on the uterus in ovariectomized mice. *J Bone Miner Metab* 27:673-681.

[328] Trivedi R, Kumar A, Gupta V, Kumar S, Nagar GK, Romero JR, Dwivedi AK, Chattopadhyay N (2009) Effects of Egb 761 on bone mineral density, bone microstructure, and osteoblast function: Possible roles of quercetin and kaempferol. *Mol Cell Endocrinol* 302:86-91.

[329] Sharan K, Mishra JS, Swarnkar G, Siddiqui JA, Khan K, Kumari R, Rawat P, Maurya R, Sanyal S, Chattopadhyay N (2011) A novel quercetin analogue from a medicinal plant promotes peak bone mass achievement and bone healing after injury and exerts an anabolic effect on osteoporotic bone: the role of aryl hydrocarbon receptor as a mediator of osteogenic action. *J Bone Miner Res* 26:2096-2111.

[330] Liang W, Luo Z, Ge S, Li M, Du J, Yang M, Yan M, Ye Z, Luo Z (2011) Oral administration of quercetin inhibits bone loss in rat model of diabetic osteopenia. *Eur J Pharmacol* 670:317-324.

[331] Horcajada-Molteni MN, Crespy V, Coxam V, Davicco MJ, Remesy C, Barlet JP (2000) Rutin inhibits ovariectomy-induced osteopenia in rats. *J Bone Miner Res* 15:2251-2258.

[332] Gu Q, Cai Y, Huang C, Shi Q, Yang H (2012) Curcumin increases rat mesenchymal stem cell osteoblast differentiation but inhibits adipocyte differentiation. *Pharmacogn Mag* 8:202-208.

[333] Moran JM, Roncero-Martin R, Rodriguez-Velasco FJ, Calderon-Garcia JF, Rey-Sanchez P, Vera V, Canal-Macias ML, Pedrera-Zamorano JD (2012) Effects of curcumin on the proliferation and mineralization of human osteoblast-like cells: implications of nitric oxide. *Int J Mol Sci 13*:16104-16118.

[334] Ozaki K, Kawata Y, Amano S, Hanazawa S (2000) Stimulatory effect of curcumin on osteoclast apoptosis. *Biochem Pharmacol* 59:1577-1581.

[335] Bharti AC, Takada Y, Aggarwal BB (2004) Curcumin (diferuloylmethan) inhibits receptor activator of NF-kappa B ligand-induced NF-kappa B activation in osteoclast precursors and suppresses osteoclastogenesis. *J Immunol* 172:5940-5947.

[336] Adams BK, Ferstl EM, Davis MC, Herold M, Kurtkaya S, Camalier RF, Hollingshead MG, Kaur G, Sausville EA, Rickles FR, Snyder JP, Liotta DC, Shoji M (2004) Synthesis and biological evaluation of novel curcumin analogs as anti-cancer and anti-angiogenesis agents. *Bioorgan Med Chem* 12:3871-3883.

[337] Kasinski AL, Du Y, Thomas SL, Zhao J, Sun S-Y, Khuri FR, Wang C-Y, Shoji M, Sun A, Snyder JP, Liotta D, Fu H (2008) *Mol Pharmacol* 74:654-661.

[338] Sun A, Lu YJ, Hu H, Shoji M, Liotta DC, Snyder JP (2009) Curcumin analog cytotoxicity against breast cancer cells: exploitation of a redox-dependent mechanism. *Bioorgan Med Chem Lett* 19:6627-6631.

[339] Yamaguchi M, Moore TW, Sun A, Snyder JP, Shoji M (2012) Novel curcumin analogue UBS109 potently stimulates osteoblastogenesis and suppresses

osteoclastogenesis: involvement in Smad activation and NF-κB inhibition. *Integr Biol* 4:905-913.

[340] Guo F, Yamashita M, Zhang Q, Zhou Q, Chen D, Reynolds DG, Awad HA, Yanoso L, Zhao L, Schwarz EM, Zhang YE, Boyce BF, Xing L (2008) Ubiquitin ligase Smurf1 mediates tumor necrosis factor-induced systemic bone loss by promoting proteasomal degradation of bone morphogenetic signaling proteins. *J Biol Chem* 283:23084-92.

[341] Yamaguchi M, Weitzmann MN (2012) The intact strontium ranelate complex stimulates osteoblastogenesis and suppresses osteoclastogenesis by antagonizing NF-κB activation. *Mol Cell Biochem* 359: 399-407.

[342] Oh S, Kyung TW, Choi HS (2008) Curcumin inhibits osteoclastogenesis by decreasing receptor activator of nuclear factor-kappaB ligand (RANKL) in bone marrow stromal cells. *Mol Cells* 30:486-489.

[343] Folwarczna J, Zych M, Trzeciak HI (2010) Effects of curcumin on the skeletal system in rats. *Pharmacol Rep* 62:900-909.

[344] Hussan F, Ibraheem NG, Kamarudin TA, Shuid AN, Soelaiman IN, Othman F (2012) Curcumin protects against ovariectomy-induced bone changes in rat model. *Evid Based Complement Alternat Med* 2012:174916. doi: 10.1155/2012/174916. Epub 2012 Sep 25.

[345] Hie M, Yamazaki M, Tsukamoto I (2009) Curcumin suppresses increased bone resorption by inhibiting osteoclastogenesis in rats with streptozotocin-induced diabetes. *Eur J Pharmacol* 621:1-9.

[346] Zhou T, Chen D, Li Q, Sun X, Song Y, Wang C (2012) Curcumin inhibits inflammatory response and bone loss during experimental periodontitis in rats. *Acta Odontol Scand* 71:349-356.

[347] Suzuki T, Nakayama H, Yamaguchi M (1997) Effect of wasabi leafstalk (*Wasabia japonica* MATSUM.) extract on bone metabolism in mouse calvaria tissue culture. *Food Sci Technol Int Tokyo* 3: 366-369.

[348] Suzuki T, Yamaguchi M (1999) Characterization of stimulatory effect of wasabi leafstalk (*Wasabia japonica* MATSUM.) extract on bone calcification in mouse calvaria tissue culture. *Food Sci Technol Res* 5: 304-307.

[349] Park JB (2013) The effects of fulvestrant, an estrogen receptor antagonists, on the proliferation, differentiation and mineralization of osteoprecursor cells. *Mol Med Reports* 7:555-558.

[350] Suzuki M, Yamaguchi M (2003) Stimulatory effect of wasabi leafstalk extract (*Wasabia japonica* MATSUM.) on bone calcification: Interaction with bone anabolic factors in mouse calvaria tissue *in vitro*. *Food Sci Technol Res* 9: 87-90.

[351] Suzuki T, Yamaguchi M (1999) Anabolic effect of wasabi leafstalk (*Wasabia japonica* MATSUM.) extract on bone metabolism in rats. *Food Sci Technol Res* 5: 61-63.

[352] Yamaguchi M, Ma ZJ, Suzuki T (2003) Anabolic effect of wasabi leafstalk (*Wasabia japonica* MATSUM.) extract on bone components in the femoral-diaphyseal and -metaphyseal tissues of aged female rats *in vitro* and *in vivo*. *J Health Sci* 49: 123-128.

[353] Yamaguchi M, Uchiyama S, Tsukamoto Y (2002) Stimulatory effect on menaquinone-7 on bone formation in elderly female rat femoral tissues in vitro: Preventive of bone deterioration with aging. *Int J Mol Med* 10:729-733.

[354] Suzuki T, Yamaguchi M (2004) Purification of active component in wasabi leafstalk (*Wasabia japonica* MATSUM) extract in stimulating bone calcification *in vitro*. *J Health Sci* 50: 483-490.

[355] Yamaguchi M (2012) Bone anabolic effect of wasabi leafstalk components: its related phytochemical *p*-hydroxycinnamic acid prevents osteoporosis. *Open Access Scientific Reports* 1: 194 (2012). doi.10.4172/scientificreports.19.

[356] Yamaguchi M, Hamamoto R, Uchiyama S, Ishiyama K, Hashimoto K (2006) Anabolic effects of bee pollen *Cistus ladaniferus* extract on bone components in the femoral-diaphyseal and –metaphyseal tissues of rats *in vitro* and *in vivo*. *J Health Sci* 52: 43-49.

[357] Yamaguchi M, Uchiyama S, Nakagawa T (2007) Anabolic effects of bee pollen *Cistus ladaniferus* extract in osteoblastic MC3T3-E1 cells *in vitro*. *J Health Sci 53,* 625-629.

[358] Hamamoto R, Ishiyama K, Yamaguchi M (2006) Inhibitory effects of bee pollen *Cistus ladaniferus* extract on bone resorption in femoral tissues and osteoclast-like cell formation in bone marrow cells in vitro. *J Health Sci* 52, 268-275.

[359] Hidaka S, Okamoto Y, Uchiyama S, Nakatsuma A, Hashimoto K, Ohnishi ST, Yamaguchi M (2006) Royal Jelly prevents osteoporosis in rats: Beneficial effects in ovariectomy model and in bone tissue culture model. Based Complement *Alternat Med* 3: 339-348.

[360] Hamamoto R, Ishiyama K, Hashimoto K, Yamaguchi M (2006) Characterization of the active component in bee pollen *Cistus ladaniferus* extract in stimulating bone calcification and in inhibiting bone resorption *in vitro*. *J Health Sci* 52: 607-612.

[361] Yamaguchi M, Uchiyama S, Nakagawa T (2007) Preventive effects of bee pollen *Cistus ladaniferus* extract on bone loss in ovariectomized rats *in vivo*. *J Health Sci* 53: 571-575.

[362] Yamaguchi M, Hamamoto R, Uchiyama S, Ishiyama K, Hashimoto K (2007) Preventive effects of bee pollen *Cistus ladaniferus* extract on bone loss in streptozotocin-diabetic rats *in vivo*. *J Health Sci* 53: 190-195.

This book was reviewed by Dr. Noriaki Shimokawa, Associate Professor, in Department of Integrative Physiology, Gunnma University Graduate School of Medicine, Maebashi, Japan, and Dr. Tomiyasu Murata, Associate Professor, in Department of Phramaceutical Sciences, Meijo University, Nagoya, Japan.

Index

C

J

K

L

M

N

O

P

Q

R

S

T

U

V

W

X

Y

Z